Smoking - Prevention, Cessation and Health Effects

Edited by Li Ping Wong and Victor Hoe

Published in London, United Kingdom

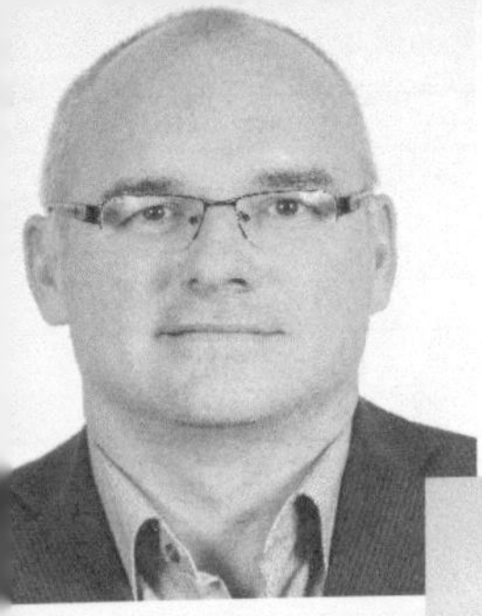
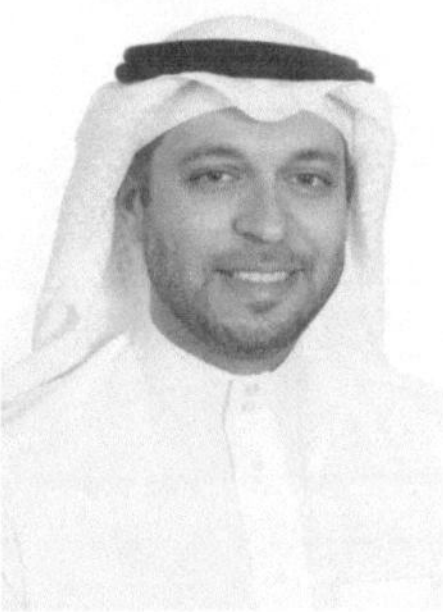
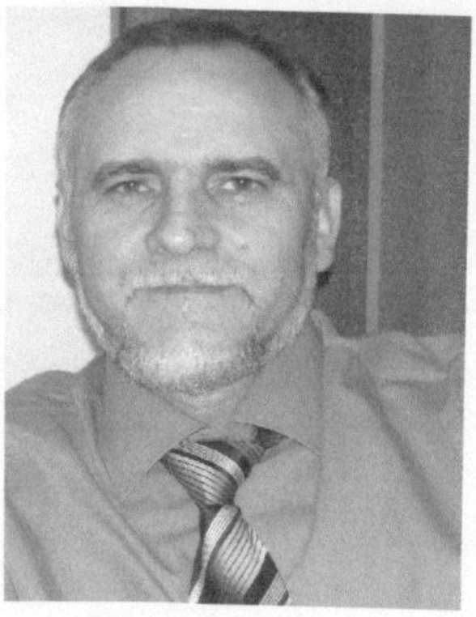
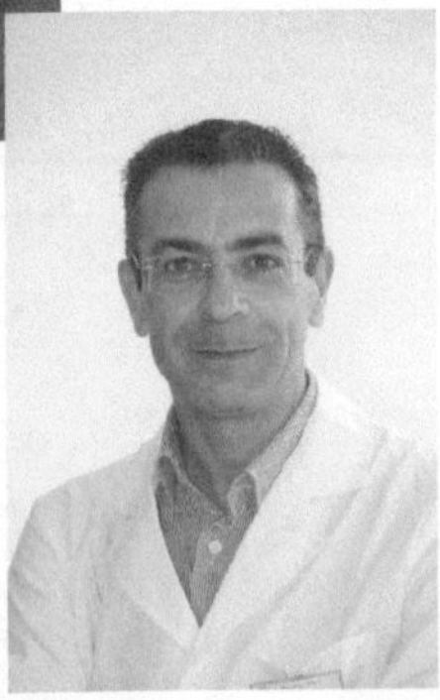
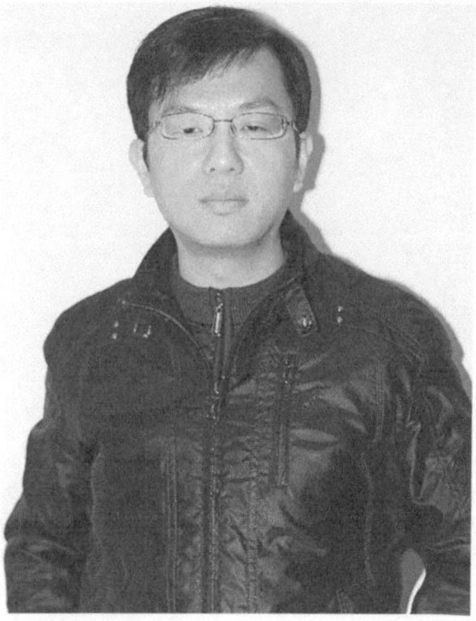
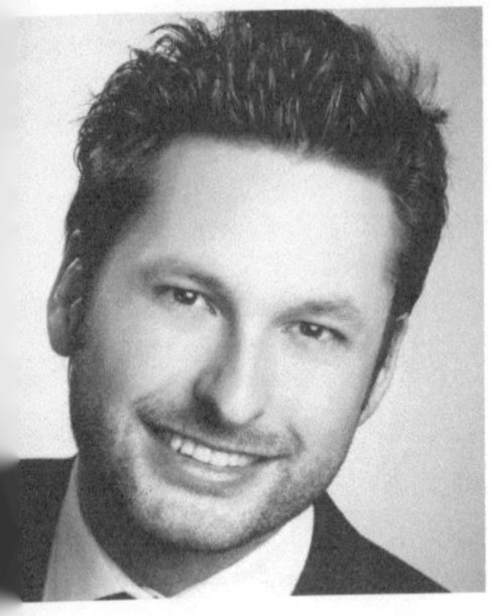
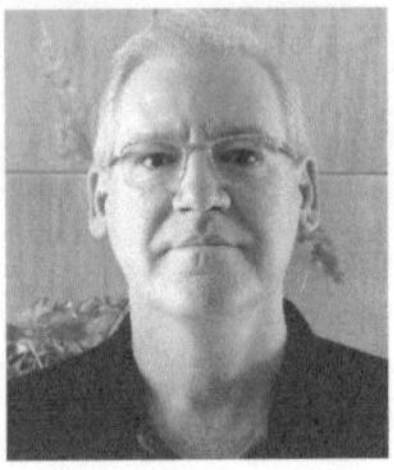

IntechOpen

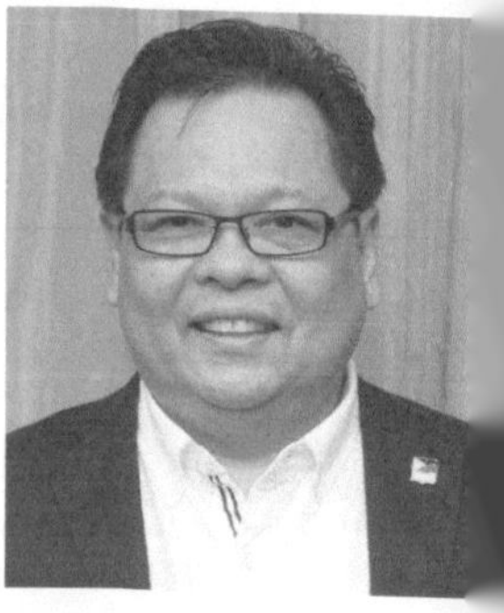
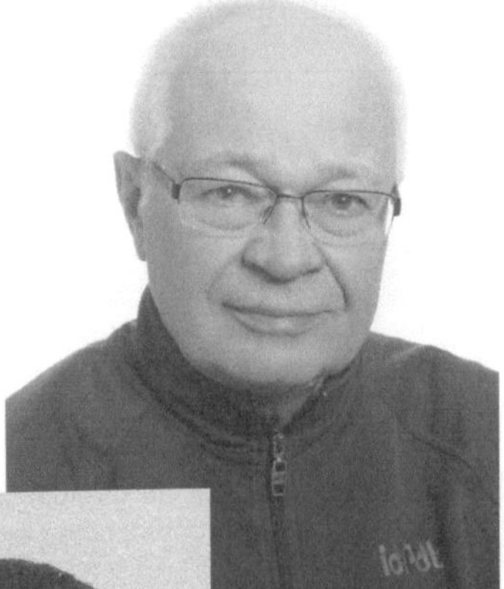
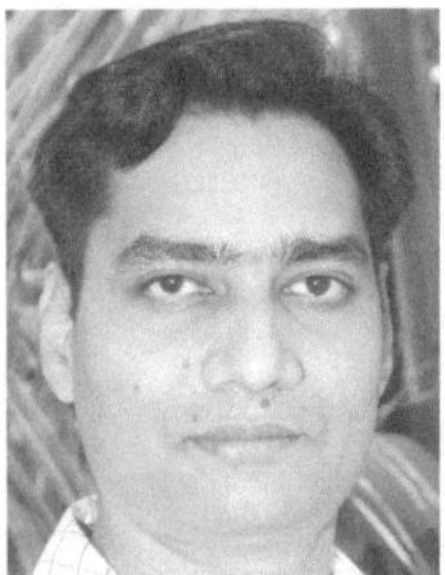
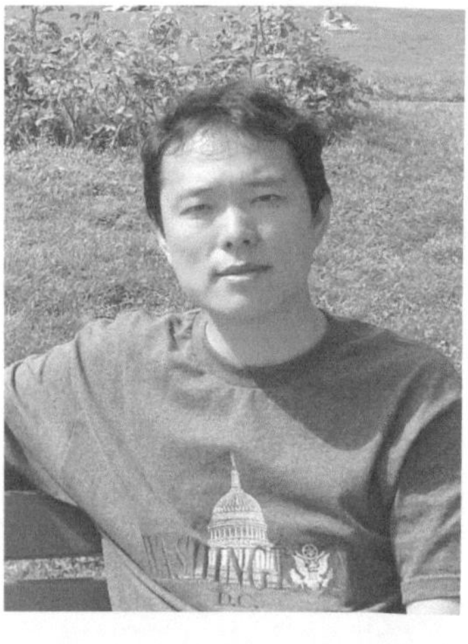
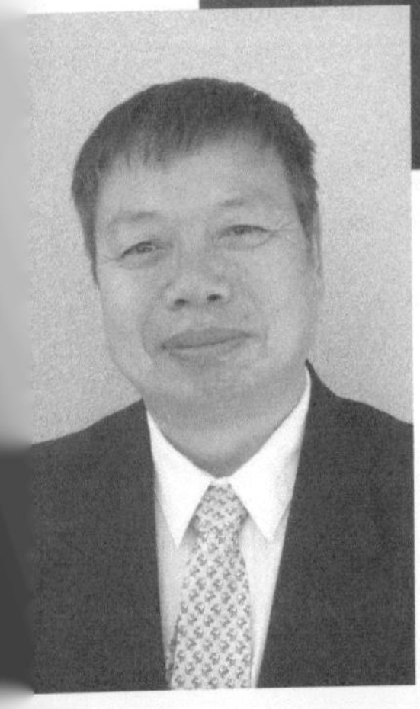
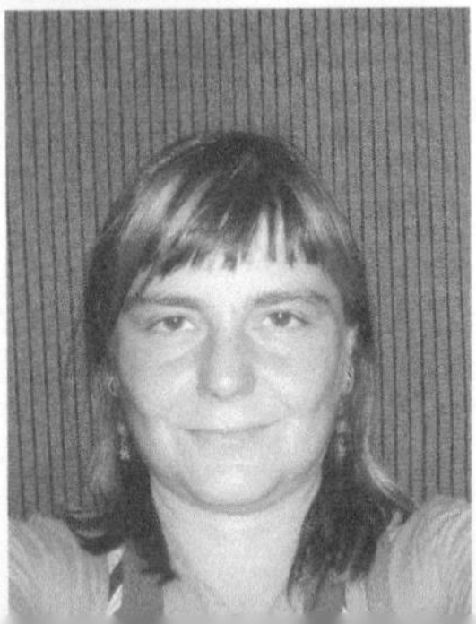

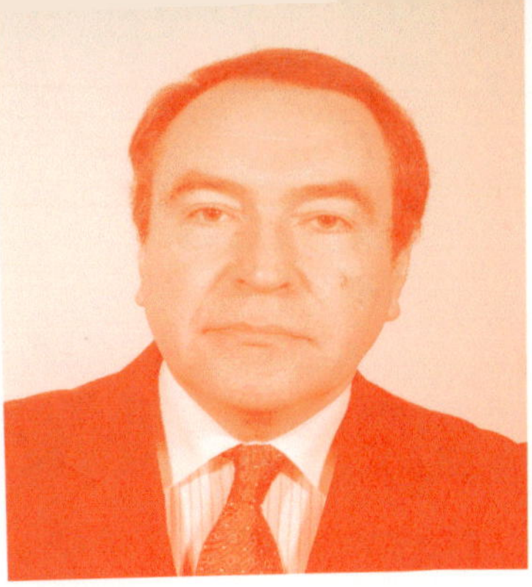

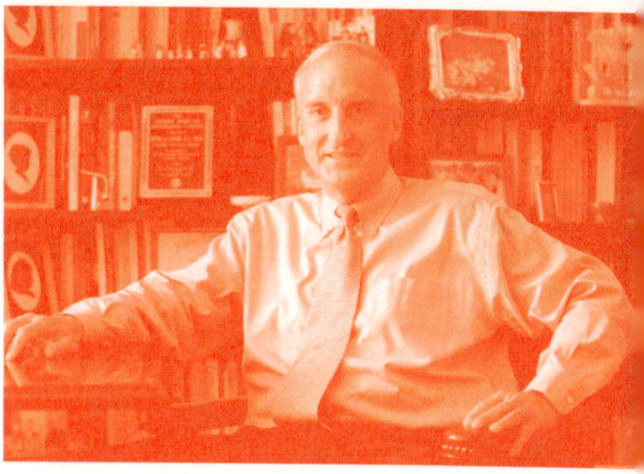

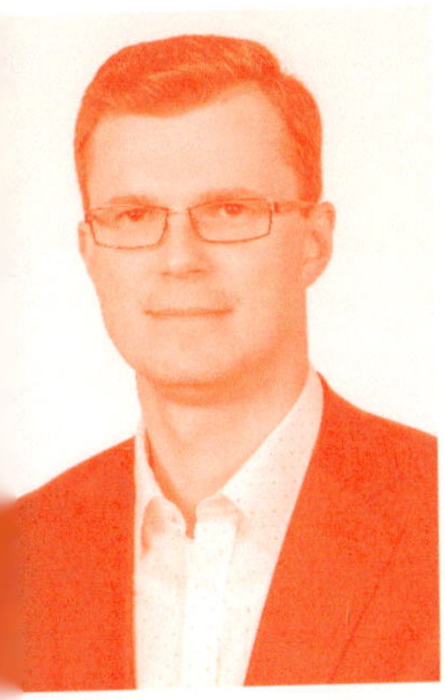

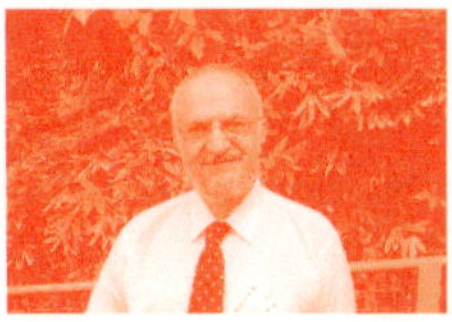

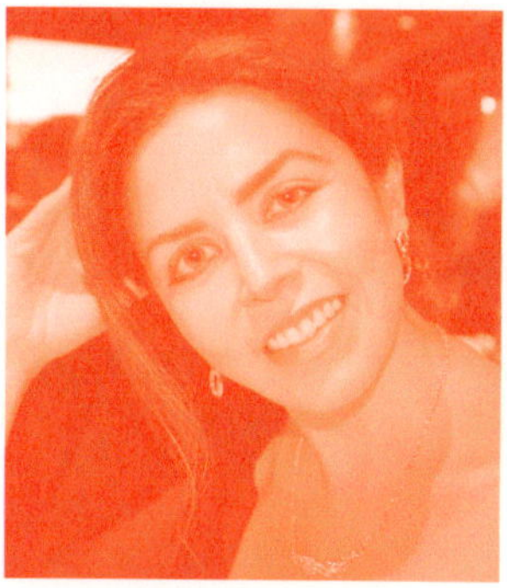

Supporting open minds since 2005

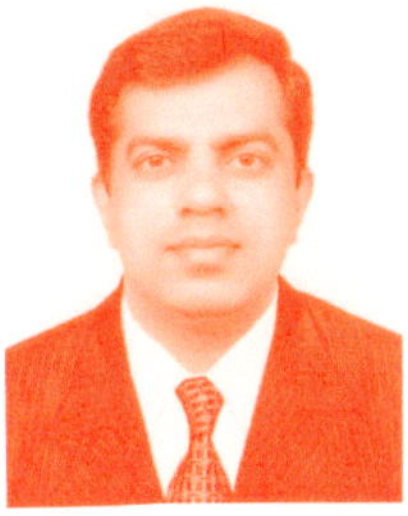

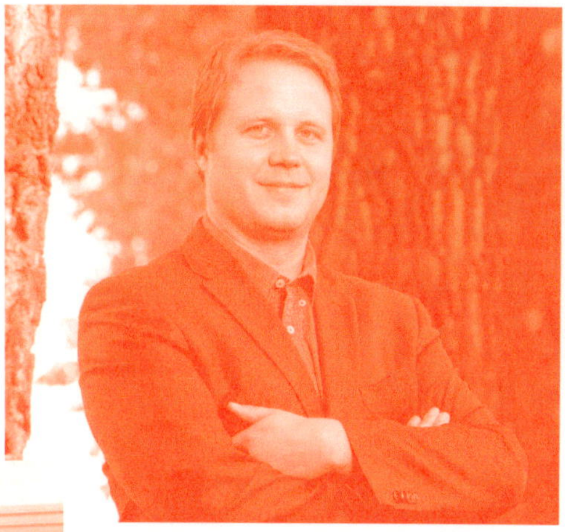

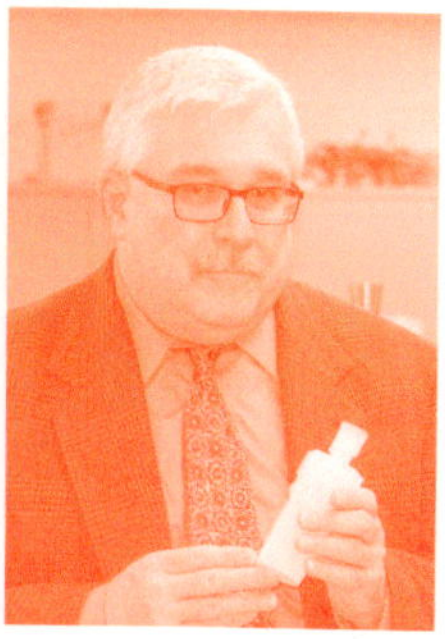

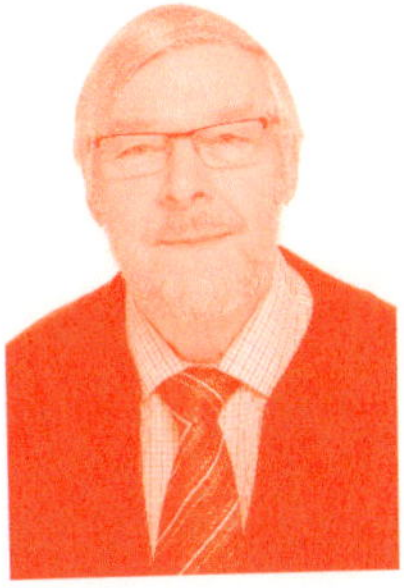

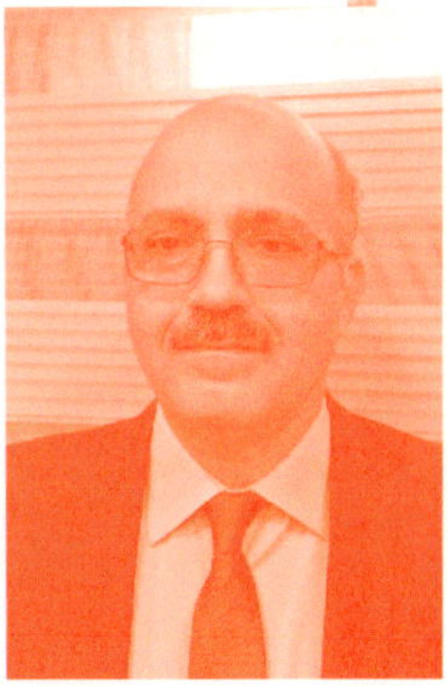

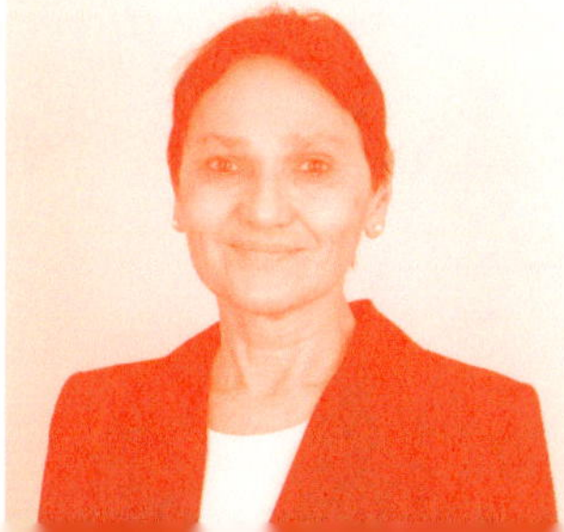

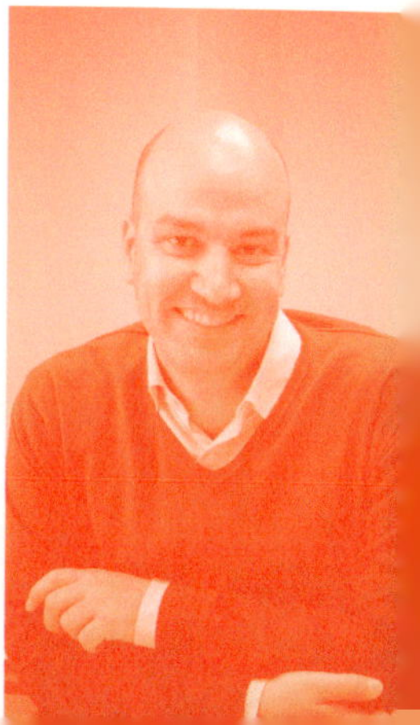

Smoking - Prevention, Cessation and Health Effects
http://dx.doi.org/10.5772/intechopen.77769
Edited by Li Ping Wong and Victor Hoe

Contributors
Narendra Maddu, Azim Chowdhury, Linda Tang, Ignatio Madanhire, Charles Mbohwa, Xiu Liu

First published in London, United Kingdom, 2019 by IntechOpen
IntechOpen is the global imprint of INTECHOPEN LIMITED, registered in England and Wales, registration number: 11086078, The Shard, 25th floor, 32 London Bridge Street
London, SE19SG - United Kingdom
Printed in Croatia

British Library Cataloguing-in-Publication Data
A catalogue record for this book is available from the British Library

Additional hard and PDF copies can be obtained from orders@intechopen.com

Smoking - Prevention, Cessation and Health Effects
Edited by Li Ping Wong and Victor Hoe
p. cm.
Print ISBN 978-1-78923-879-2
Online ISBN 978-1-78923-880-8
eBook (PDF) ISBN 978-1-78984-318-7

Meet the editors

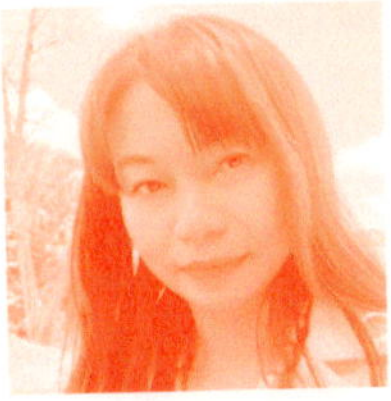

Li Ping Wong, PhD, is a professor in the Department of Social and Preventive Medicine, Faculty of Medicine, University of Malaya, Malaysia. She earned her PhD in Medical Science (Epidemiology) from the University of Malaya. She takes part in the faculty's research methodology, epidemiology, and biostatistical teaching both at undergraduate and graduate levels. Her current research interests and more than 120 publications are in the areas of social epidemiology and behavioral medicine. She has worked on a series of articles concerning risky behaviors (electronic cigarettes use, antisocial behaviors, and unprotected sexual intercourse), public health and preventive behaviors (H1N1 influenza, cervical cancer, human papillomavirus, and HIV infection), behavioral responses to emerging infectious diseases (2009 influenza H1N1 and Zika), and sexual reproductive health (midlife crisis, dysmenorrheal, and premenstrual syndromes).

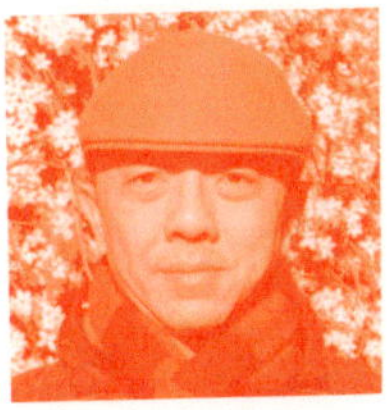

Prof. Dr. Victor Hoe is an occupational physician with a practice in the University Malaya Medical Centre and teaches at the Department of Social and Preventive Medicine, Faculty of Medicine, University of Malaya. He has worked with ExxonMobil, Department of Occupational Safety and Health, Social Security Organization, National Institute of Occupational Safety and Health, Hospital Kuala Lumpur, Pengkalan Hulu Health Clinic, and Ministry of Health Malaysia. He has been involved in various research projects, including being part of the multinational research project Cultural and Psychosocial Influences on Disability, which involved researchers from 18 countries, and the cohort study on clustering of lifestyle risk factors and understanding their association with stress on health and wellbeing among school teachers in Malaysia (CLUSTer). He was also involved in various consultancy projects on occupational health and environmental impact assessment. He has published 38 papers and abstracts in peer-reviewed journals. He is the editor of *BMC Musculoskeletal Disorders*, *Medical Journal of Malaysia*, and *Journal of Health and Translational Medicine* (JUMMEC). He is currently council member for the Academy of Occupational and Environmental Medicine Malaysia and the College of Public Health Medicine-Academy of Medicine Malaysia, and an executive member for the Malaysian Medical Association Wilayah Branch, the Asia-Pacific Academic Consortium for Public Health, and the International Commission for Occupational Health National Secretary for Malaysia.

Contents

Preface

Tobacco smoking is one of the greatest causes of mortality in the world. It is a dangerous lifestyle choice that results in increased risk of premature death and serious morbidities. Although the adverse health effects from tobacco usage are well documented, this book provides a detailed compilation of health risks associated with tobacco smoking and its impact. Environmental smoke causes the same serious conditions as active smoking. The implication of passive smoking and serious health implications for both children and adults are highlighted to increase knowledge of the health effects of second-hand smoke. Therefore, apart from physical health risk, social health risk and the environmental impact of smoking are illustrated to create societal recognition of the dangers of smoking and support for a smoke-free environment.

Electronic cigarettes are marketed as a smoking cessation product and a healthier alternative to smoked tobacco. The issue of electronic cigarettes is one of the most controversial topics in public health. The positive health effects described in this book are that electronic cigarettes can help individuals quit smoking, they are healthier than smoking, and they have no smoke or second-hand smoke exposure. However, the health effects of electronic cigarettes have been a contentious topic in the scientific community. Some evidence suggests that electronic cigarette use may facilitate smoking cessation, but definitive data are lacking. Thus, this book also presents a collection of ideas and research findings of the role of electronic cigarettes in the prevention and cessation strategies of smoking. This book is beneficial as a guidance for people who want to quit smoking with the aid of electronic cigarettes and to understand their health impacts and dangers. The empirical evidence of the adverse health impacts of electronic smoking is described. Electronic cigarette laws and regulation are also discussed in this book.

Li Ping Wong and Victor Hoe
Department of Social and Preventive Medicine,
University of Malaya,
Malaysia

Chapter 1

Impact of Smoking in a Tobacco-Growing Developing Country: A Review

Ignatio Madanhire and Charles Mbohwa

Abstract

The chapter reviews the impact of smoking on a developing country whose economy heavily depends on growing tobacco. Other than the pollution of the air caused by tobacco smoke, large areas of forestry land is destroyed, and huge losses are incurred due to perennial veldt fires. These would damage properties, flora, and fauna, and in some cases human life is lost. Public health bill is increasing annually to carter for smoking-related cancer which has become the major killer disease ahead of HIV/AIDS in the country. The levying of excise duty on cigarette sales to control tobacco smoking is not deterrent enough. There has been a marked increase in smoking by the youth of school-going age, and this risk behavior has been attributed to excessive exposure to intense advertising by the tobacco industry. Weak legal framework has not done enough to enforce tobacco smoking control, prohibition of public smoking, and sale of tobacco to the under-aged individuals. It was established that the common view that the thriving tobacco industry is responsible for key economic exports does not promote initiatives to reduce cigarette smoking.

Keywords: smoking, cigarettes, control, pollution, health, environment

1. Introduction

Cigarette smoking habit is normally started at an early age, and it continues into one's adult life [1]. According to prior studies, if one starts smoking, it will be difficult for one to stop the practice. Among those who continue to smoke throughout their lives, it is estimated that about half are expected to die from some smoking-related causes [2, 3]. It is for this reason that adolescents and school-aged children should be a primary focus for all intervention strategies [1, 2]. There is a need to put in place initiatives and strategic alliances to effectively address the negative impact of tobacco and to encourage and support children to lead healthy and active lives free from tobacco smoking [1].

It is estimated that, of the 6.6 billion people in the world, 1.3 billion are smokers and 1 billion of these are males [2]. By the year 2030, tobacco will be the single biggest cause of death worldwide causing more deaths than HIV, malaria, tuberculosis, maternal mortality, automobile crashes, homicides, and suicides combined [1, 3]. It is also estimated that tobacco-related diseases will account for 11% of all deaths that will occur in developing countries by 2025. So far, no other consumer products have come close to inflicting this degree of harm on the world community [2].

IntechOpen

2. Background

Zimbabwe has a long history of growing tobacco. In 2012, the country was the top tobacco-producing nation in Africa, while in 2013 it was the sixth largest tobacco producer in the world [3, 4]. According to Zimbabwe's tobacco industry and marketing board, 98% of Zimbabwe's tobacco is exported. Thus tobacco is the country's largest foreign currency earner accounting for 10–43% of the country's gross domestic product [5].

Tobacco industry is a major source of employment for the population. There are currently over 90,000 tobacco farmers. Tobacco growing is given top priority despite widespread food insecurity and environmental degradation resulting thereof. As a result farmers are highly incentivized to grow tobacco than grain food crops [4, 5].

The country recently joined other countries in the Framework Convention on Tobacco Control (FCTC), which obligates nations to implement a variety of tobacco control measures [3]. These entail the requirement for member countries to adopt and implement measures that address tobacco control in three domains—tobacco demand reduction, tobacco supply reduction, and protecting the environment [5, 6]. It was observed that Zimbabwe has implemented several measures aimed at reducing tobacco demand, but very few aimed at reducing tobacco supply or protecting the environment.

3. Tobacco smoking trends

The smoking prevalence among females in Zimbabwe is about 5%, and for men it is much higher at 33%. This observation reflects the growing popularity of smoking among males in the country. This demonstrates the need for tobacco control in the country [1, 2]. The country has a few tobacco control measures and one national tobacco control law, Statutory Instrument 264 of 2002 [3]. The smoking of cigarettes is associated with negative social, health, and economic consequences, which can affect both smokers and non-smokers alike.

It has been observed that smoking-related diseases in African countries are lower than international standards. The increase in smoking prevalence suggests a looming epidemic of smoking-related diseases. Information on tobacco use among young people is not readily available for most developing countries like Zimbabwe, where the last survey was conducted 10 years ago [1, 3]. Thus if the effort on tobacco control is to succeed globally, the progress has to be equally made in Zimbabwe, and the impact of intervention has to be closely monitored and evaluated.

Current interventions entail making it a mandatory requirement to put health warnings on cigarette packages, designating smoke-free zones in public settings, and all cigarette sales are levied at 60%. While there are laws to prevent tobacco sales to minors, the youths from both urban and rural settings have reported that they have easy access to cigarettes [3, 4, 6]. Efforts being made to send anti-smoking messages to the youths are being diluted by massive advertising by tobacco industry portraying "positive" images of cigarette smoking. Urban residents are always exposed to contradicting messages as they have ready access to media channels such televisions, newspapers, and magazines [3, 5]. Billboards are erected, and sporting events such as soccer matches are used to promote cigarette smoking. Brazil, which is the world's top tobacco producer, managed to reduce tobacco use by 50%, without affecting its revenue coming from exports. Tobacco control measures that target internal tobacco use cause little conflict with export profits. This example suggests that Zimbabwe may also be able to implement tobacco control at home with insignificant impact on exports [4].

The FCTC has been slow to agree on a coherent and effective policy to support economically viable alternatives to tobacco growing and protecting the environment.

4. Economic impact

Zimbabwe is the largest grower of tobacco in Africa and the sixth largest grower in the world. Tobacco plays a big role in the Zimbabwean economy. According to statistics by the UN's food and agriculture organization, tobacco is the Zimbabwe's largest export commodity— and it accounts for nearly 10% of GDP as shown by activity in **Figure 1** [7, 8].

Tobacco production in the country reached its peak of 217 million kilograms in 2014 as shown in **Table 1**. In 2015, 54% of Zimbabwe's tobacco exports was sold to China [8, 9].

Cigarette consumption per capita is the total annual number of cigarette sticks consumed divided by the total adult population aged 15 years and above in the country. **Figure 2** shows that the major declines in cigarette consumption occurred in 1982, 1984, 1992, and 2005–2008 [8, 9]. During 1982 and 1992, the consumption declined due to the occurrence of drought in the country, and consumers diverted their attention from purchasing more cigarettes to buying food stuff for themselves and their families. In 2004 up to 2008, there was an economic decline, and the Zimbabwean dollar was depreciating in the hyperinflationary environment in the country [8]. A decline in the economy affected agricultural output which in turn affected the manufacturing industries adversely in terms of reduced output and resultant company closures. The closing down of companies led to an increase in the number of unemployed individuals with little disposable income, which led to a decrease in consumption. In 2009–2011, the country introduced a multicurrency system, and there was an increase in consumption. From 2011 to 2015, **Figure 2** shows a decline in consumption that was influenced by an increase in excise tax on retail prices for all cigarette tobacco sales which led to reduced demand [10, 11].

In previous studies, it was observed that a positive price elasticity of cigarettes implied that increasing tax on the tobacco cigarettes would only raise tax revenue and not necessarily reduce the demand for the consumption of the product [3, 4].

Considering the addictive behavior associated with the product, the demand for cigarettes does not follow the essential laws of economics and the theory of demand [9]. Thus the cigarettes being an addictive product, there is no demand influence on the change in price of the commodity. Instead peer networks have a positive and significant influence on smoking intensity and participation, compared to excise tax and tobacco control policies that may be introduced by the government of the day [10].

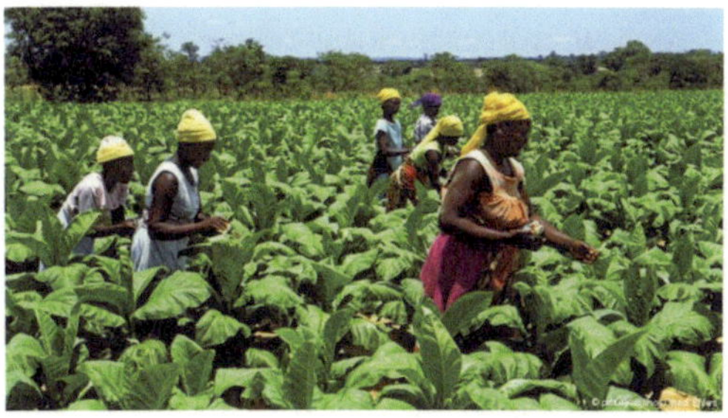

Figure 1.
Tobacco field (ZTB 2018).

Year	Tobacco production (million kg)
2004	69
2005	73
2008	48
2010	59
2011	124
2012	144
2013	167
2014	217
2015	189
2016	195

Table 1.
Tobacco production trend (ZIMSTAT, 2017).

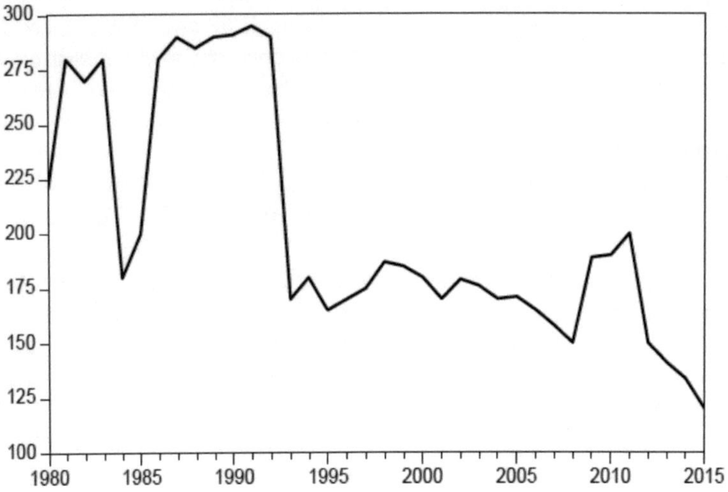

Figure 2.
Cigarette consumption per capita [14].

5. Social impact

According to WHO report in 2018, smoking is considered as a preventable cause of premature death in developed countries, whereas smoking epidemic in developing countries is now becoming even more popular and accepted as a societal norm [4, 6]. These countries mostly concentrate on malnutrition and infectious diseases, and they give low priority to tobacco cigarette smoking-related issues.

In the country, the government fears that a levy increase on cigarette sales and other proven cost-effective tobacco control measures would harm its economy in terms of revenue, job, and income losses. Despite that the demand for cigarettes is inelastic, Zimbabwe is one of the countries that have the lowest excise tax on cigarettes in Africa at 40% (**Figure 3**), and this is way below the recommended WHO excise tax rate of 75–80%, which could effectively reduce demand [5, 7]. Thus hiking excise tax rate is an effective measure to reduce cigarette smoking as well as reduce tobacco-related social costs [10].

It was observed that the majority of smokers become addicted when they are still teenagers [12]. Among other reasons, the youths smoke for them to look mature, to

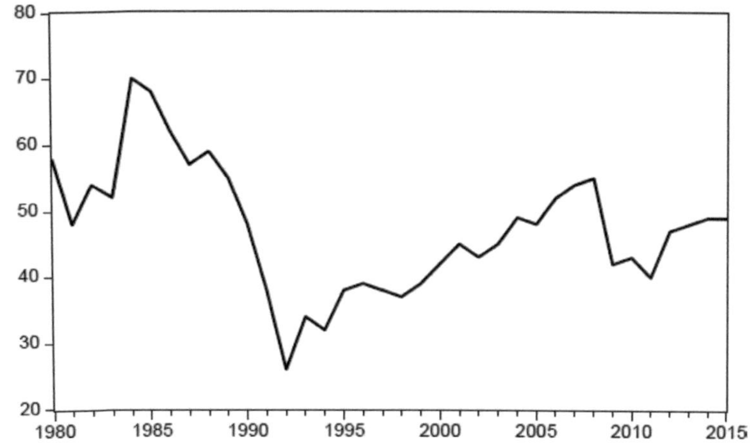

Figure 3.
Excise tax in Zimbabwe (%) (ZIMSTAT, 2017).

experiment, and to be like their friends. This brings out the fact that smoking also provides a social reward by making the consumer feel like they are part of a group, which provides a sense of comfort and acceptance [13].

The consumption of cigarettes is increasing in the country. Adults smoke when they experience mounting stress and pressures due to personal and economic challenges. They would smoke in order to feel relaxed and get energy to get over their problems. Others smoke because smoking makes them feel good about themselves and it gives them a sense of pleasure [9].

Provision of educational programs in the school curriculum may be necessary to educate the youth on the short- and long-term effects of cigarette smoking. It may also be necessary to introduce effective warning labels on all tobacco cigarette products. The government can introduce a system that sends text messages to every individual using cellular networks stating the bad effects of smoking and encouraging people to stop smoking [1]. It could also provide cessation programs and medication to smokers to help them quit and provide medical education advising smokers that quitting is cheaper than treating smoking-related illnesses.

6. Environmental impact

The tobacco industry damages the environment in ways that go far beyond the effects of the smoke that cigarettes put into the air. Tobacco growing, manufacturing of cigarettes, and process of delivering products to retailers all have environmental impacts that may include deforestation, the use of fossil fuels, and dumping or leaking of cigarette waste products into the natural environment [14]. The whole life cycle from growing tobacco plants to the disposal of cigarette butts negatively impacts the environment. The ecological impacts of tobacco are serious cause for concern, especially in a tobacco-growing country like Zimbabwe [3].

6.1 Cigarette butts and the environment

6.1.1 Veldt fires

Cigarette smoking in rural and commercial farming areas is considered to be the common cause of most veldt fires when smoldering butts are thrown on dry grass (**Figure 4**). The farming land destroyed by veldt fires in Zimbabwe amounted to 950,905 hectares in 2009, 1,152,413 hectares in 2010, 713,770 hectares in 2011, and 1,320,325 hectares in 2012. In this regard, veldt fires pose a serious challenge to environmental sustainability [11, 15].

Figure 5 shows that most veldt fires are caused by careless human activities such as improper disposal of cigarette stubs and burning of vegetation during land preparation (these two being the major causes). The least causes according to Forsyth et al. [12] are smoking bees and motorist who prepare fire for warming themselves in case of a vehicle breakdown at night.

The veldt fires have adverse impact on the environment especially in communal areas, where they have destroyed any damageable material. Trees, species of wildlife, farming land, livestock, human lives, and livelihoods suffer under the severe threat posed by veldt fires [2, 3]. The natural environment has suffered the destruction of fauna and flora, while the loss of property, pollution, and at times injury have been the order of the day in the human environment [11, 12]. Veldt fires also result in the decline of veldt conditions and an increase in air pollution, thereby reducing the quality of air that people would use to breathe. These fires emit millions of tons of gases and particulate matter into the air, which will have serious consequences on human health and carbon balances that contribute to global climate change [2, 4].

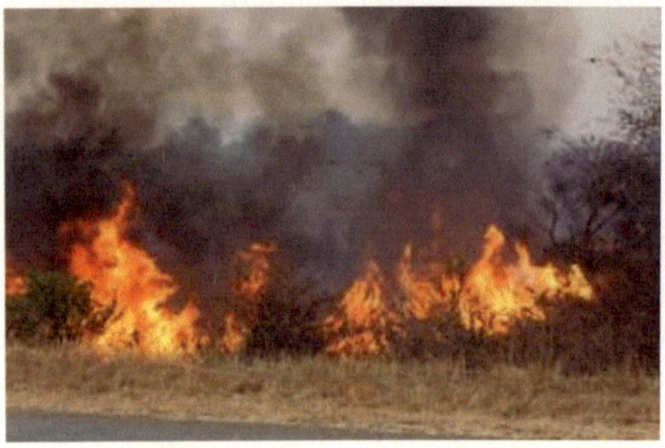

Figure 4.
Veldt fire in Karoi area, Zimbabwe.

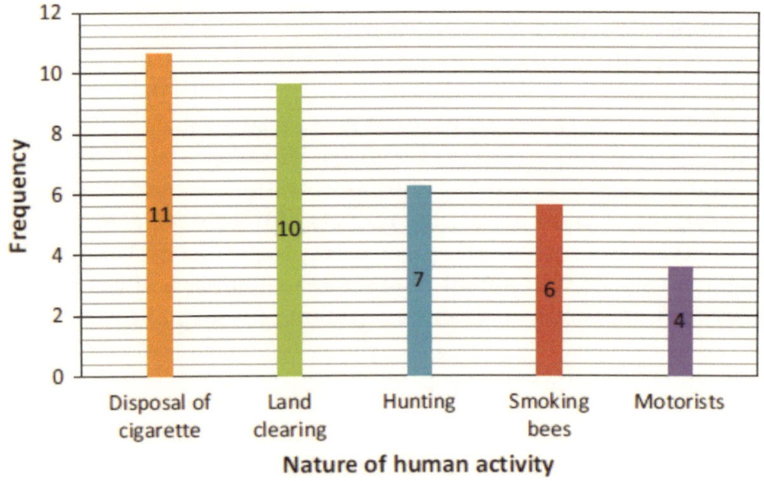

Figure 5.
Smoking topping causes of veldt fires.

If not controlled, veldt fires would give rise to unclean environment, severe environmental degradation, and diminished livelihoods [11, 12]. This would result in severe destruction of the veldt, thereby adversely affecting flora and fauna. Therefore veldt fires also pose some danger to human life since communities depend on the very degraded environment [11]. Air and water can be polluted by such veldt fires, thereby creating health hazards due to the resulting non sustainability of natural environment.

It is in this regard that there is a need to come up with sound interventions to protect, preserve, and sustain the environment. Enforcing of tobacco smoking control legislation may go a long way in reducing veldt fire incidence.

6.1.2 Water pollution

Tobacco waste is the end point in the life cycle of cigarettes, and the resulting cigarette butts are the largest single type of litter by count. Tobacco waste ends up everywhere, and it is a well-known public nuisance for many communities, especially those with few resources to remove it [12]. Cleanup and disposal are costs of tobacco consumption that are not currently borne by manufacturers, distributors, or users of tobacco products [15]. The cleanup costs of tobacco waste in the form of discarded cigarette butts are generally borne by municipalities. Cigarette butts on disposal in landfill produce further liquid wastes such as heavy metals and poisons such as arsenic that leach from butts [16].

Long after a cigarette has been extinguished, it continues to cause environmental damage in the form of non-biodegradable butts—millions of kilograms of which are discarded every year [17]. Butts are the most common item accumulating in local waste stream. Tossing a cigarette butt on the ground has become one of the most accepted forms of littering globally, and this has become a social norm for many smokers [14, 16]. The increase of butt disposal directly into the environment has been attributed to imposed restrictions on smoking in workplaces, bars, restaurants, etc. (**Figure 6**).

Toxic chemicals in cigarette butts contribute to nonpoint source pollution, when butts are carried through storm drains by rainfall and urban runoff to dams, rivers, wetlands, and even underground sources of drinking water [15, 16]. Nonpoint source pollution has harmful effects on drinking water supplies.

Studies have also shown that harmful chemicals such as nicotine, arsenic, polycyclic aromatic hydrocarbons (PAHs), and heavy metals leach from discarded tobacco butt waste and can be acutely toxic to aquatic organisms such as fish [16]. A butt may look like the end of the damage brought by a cigarette, but there is still a way to go in addressing postconsumer waste cleanup and responsible disposal [11].

6.2 Environmental tobacco smoke (ETS) pollution

Environmental tobacco smoke (ETS) could be described as the material in indoor air that originates from tobacco smoke (**Figure 7**). Breathing in ETS is known as passive smoking, secondhand smoke, or involuntary smoking [10].

Tobacco smoke consists of solid particles and gases. The solid components of tobacco smoke such as tar and nicotine make up 10%, while the gases constitutes about 90%. The major gas present in tobacco smoke is carbon monoxide. Other gases include formaldehyde, acrolein, ammonia, nitrogen oxides, pyridine, hydrogen cyanide, vinyl chloride, N-nitrosodimethylamine, and acrylonitrile. Of these, formaldehyde, N-nitrosodimethylamine, and vinyl chloride are suspected or known carcinogens in humans. Acrylonitrile has been known to cause cancer in animals [14, 16].

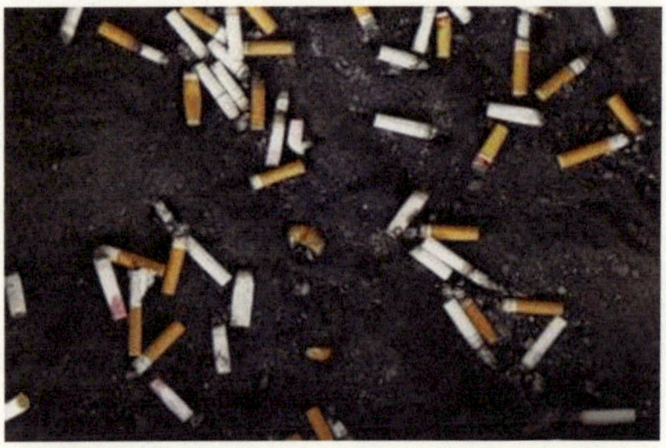

Figure 6.
Discarded cigarette stubs (Picture by: I Madanhire).

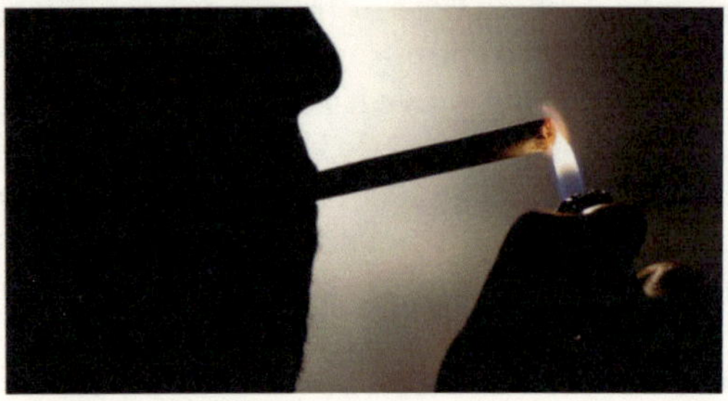

Figure 7.
Indoor smoke producing.

Environmental tobacco smoke is composed of both mainstream and sidestream smoke. ETS is diluted by the air in the room before it is inhaled and is therefore less concentrated than mainstream or sidestream smoke. Every person—both smokers and non-smokers—in a room with ETS will have similar exposure because nearly 85% of ETS in a room comes from sidestream smoke (**Figure 9**). The smoker is also exposed to mainstream smoke, but this exposure is limited to the time it takes to smoke a cigarette [6, 10]. However, exposure to ETS remains constant for the entire time spent in that room.

Exposure to ETS has been estimated in terms of "cigarette equivalents." Cigarette equivalents can be measured by determining carboxyhemoglobin levels in blood. Carboxyhemoglobin is formed in the blood when someone inhales carbon monoxide. The hemoglobin in the blood that has oxygen bound to it is called oxyhemoglobin. It is the oxyhemoglobin that carries oxygen to the tissues. However, carbon monoxide has a much stronger attraction to hemoglobin than oxygen. Thus, inhaled carbon monoxide quickly replaces the oxygen in the oxyhemoglobin and binds to the hemoglobin to form carboxyhemoglobin which can be measured [6, 7]. Various studies suggest that passive exposure to ETS over an 8-hour day is comparable to directly smoking one to three cigarettes.

While no single study can say that there is a 100% chance of health problems as a result of exposure to ETS, an association between ETS and various health conditions is considered very likely because there is:

- The proven link between heart diseases and lung cancer to active smoking

- The presence of several known carcinogens in environmental tobacco smoke

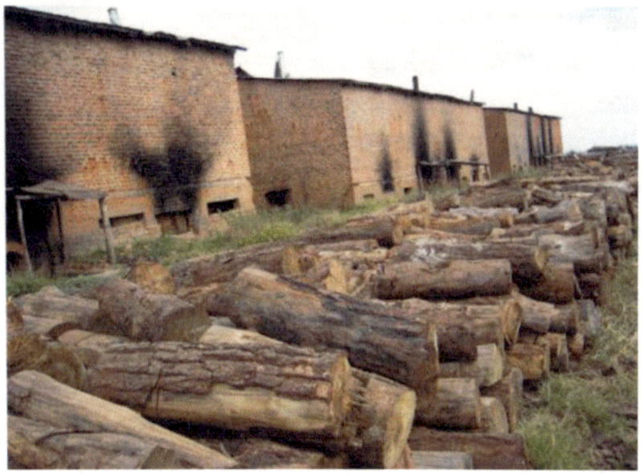

Figure 8.
Deforestation-related tobacco curing barns.

- The general acceptance that the risks of certain diseases are directly related to the amount of tobacco smoke inhaled

When evidence from various studies is combined, they indicate that exposure to ETS increases the number of lung cancers detected in non-smokers. Non-smoking co-workers of smokers have a relative risk of being affected. Non-smokers with heart disease (angina pectoris) exposed to ETS in ventilated and unventilated rooms had increased heart rates, elevated blood pressures, and increased carbon monoxide in the blood. ETS aggravates allergy symptoms. It is generally more irritating to the respiratory tract of asthmatics, and it can aggravate some asthmatic symptoms such as wheezing [3].

Many of the substances in cigarette smoke are very irritating to the eyes, throat, and respiratory mucous membranes. A high proportion of non-smokers report eye irritation, headache, nasal discomfort, cough, sore throat, or sneezing when exposed to cigarette smoke. Eye irritation seems the main symptom during passive exposure to cigarette smoke.

6.3 Deforestation

Tobacco farming is the main cause of deforestation in countries such as Zimbabwe (**Figure 8**). There is evidence of substantial, and largely irreversible, losses of trees and other plant species caused by tobacco farming that make it a particular threat to biodiversity [5].

Tobacco control efforts aimed at the protection of the environment and health of persons represent another hurdle. Deforestation is a particularly significant problem in Zimbabwe, since flue-cured tobacco requires heat to process the leaves and wood is used as a fuel supply [6].

After harvesting, tobacco is dried and cured to preserve it for storage, transport, and processing. Indigenous trees are cut down to provide fuel for the curing process and construction of curing barns as given in **Figure 8**; as a crop it is responsible for damage to ancient forests [13].

7. Smoking impact on public health

No matter how one smokes it, tobacco is dangerous to one's health. There are no safe substances in any tobacco products, from acetone and tar to nicotine and carbon monoxide. The substances one inhales do not just affect the lungs. They can affect the entire body. Tobacco smoke is incredibly harmful to human health. There is no safe way to smoke.

Cigarette smoking harms nearly every organ of the body, causes many diseases, and reduces the health of smokers in general (**Figure 9**). Quitting smoking lowers one's risk for smoking-related diseases and can add years to one's life [3]. Smoking harms nearly every organ of the body and affects a person's overall health [7]. Smoking causes diminished overall health, increased absenteeism from work, and increased healthcare utilization and cost [11].

Regardless of the widespread knowledge of the harm caused by smoking, only little success has been achieved in tobacco control initiatives. It is estimated that there are currently 3.5 million deaths a year from tobacco, and this figure is expected to rise about 10 million by 2030 [7, 10]. By that date, 70% of the deaths will be experienced in developing countries [8].

Tobacco use is distinguished from many other health problems by the presence of an aggressive, transnational tobacco industry whose goals are fundamentally incompatible with public health [2, 3]. Like other industries, the tobacco industry does not only seek to promote the use of its products and expand into new markets but also seeks to weaken strong tobacco control policies and undermine public health advocacy efforts [4].

There is a strong relationship between smoking prevalence and lung cancer patterns. Because smoking is the major cause of lung cancer and lung cancer commonly takes 20 or more years to develop, smoking prevalence is an important predictor of future lung cancer patterns [7]. Likewise, today's lung cancer patterns are a good indicator of the smoking prevalence of previous decades. When one takes up smoking, there is a greater chance of contracting cancer later in life. It can

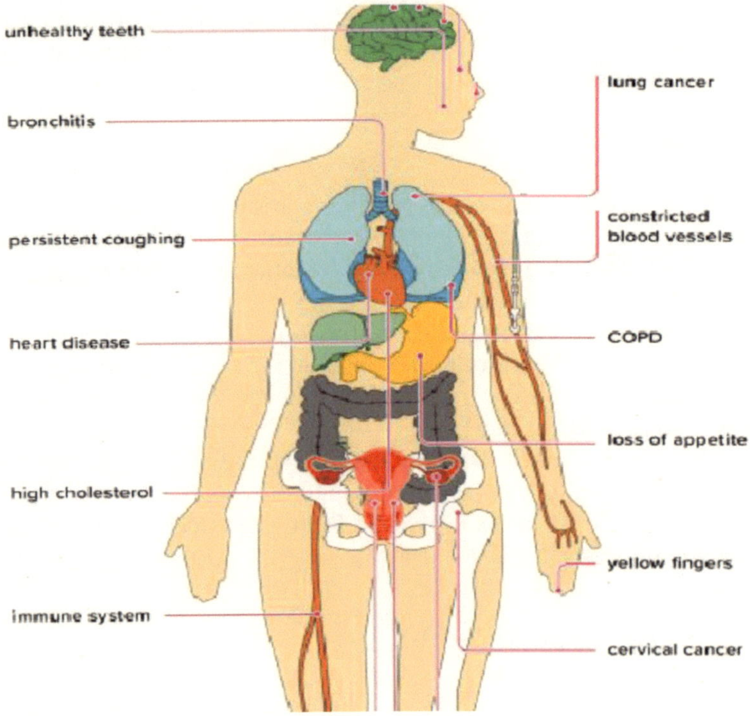

Figure 9.
Smoking effects on human body.

be assumed with accuracy that a majority of the youths that are current smokers would develop lung cancer before they reach the age of 35 years [10]. Smoking can cause lung disease by damaging the airways and the small air sacs (alveoli) found in the lungs. Lung diseases caused by smoking include chronic obstructive pulmonary disease (COPD), which includes emphysema and chronic bronchitis. If you have asthma, tobacco smoke can trigger an attack or make an attack worse [7].

There are also other diseases that are caused by smoking, such as heart diseases, strokes, and a range of respiratory diseases. Smoking causes about 80% of all deaths from COPD. Smoking damages blood vessels and can make them thicken and grow narrower. This makes the heart beat faster and one's blood pressure to go up. Clots can also form. A stroke occurs when a clot blocks the blood flow to parts of your brain, and a blood vessel in or around your brain bursts [7, 10]. Blockages caused by smoking can also reduce blood flow to your legs and skin.

Smoking can affect bone health. Women past childbearing years who smoke have weaker bones than women who never smoked. They are also at greater risk for broken bones. Smoking affects the health of your teeth and gums and can cause tooth loss [7]. Smoking causes general adverse effects on the body, including inflammation and decreased immune function.

Some effort is being made to ban smoking in public places but not at an individual level. Very few are aware of the dangers of smoke from other people's cigarettes with yet fewer in favor of banning smoking in public places. This is unmistakably a lack of knowledge on the dangers of environmental tobacco smoke to one's health [8]. During the past two or so decades, research has been undertaken worldwide to reveal the evidence on the health effects of passive smoking. These studies have concluded that passive smoking increases the chances of contracting or aggravating a range of illnesses including cardiovascular disease, lung cancer as mentioned above, asthma (particularly in children), acute irritation of the respiratory tract, bronchitis, pneumonia, and other chest illnesses in children [10].

One huge problem that cannot be overshadowed by the economic use of tobacco is its increased use by young people and the long-term effects to their health [1].

8. Highlights on smoking in Zimbabwe

The current smokers could have been enticed into smoking by associating with smokers or frequenting places where smoking is a common practice like beer halls and clubs. Surprisingly though, not many smokers are in favor of banning smoking in public places, with less than half saying they are in favor [1]. There are difficulties as some of the current smokers try to quit smoking in recent past, with no success.

However smokers often do not take into serious consideration the long-term consequences of smoking behaviors. For youths, the risks of tobacco use are perceived to be remote and are outweighed by what they see as the immediate benefits [5]. They tend to underestimate the addictiveness of nicotine and the difficulties associated with quitting; they believe it is easier for young people to quit than adults.

Due to the proven association between high-risk behaviors like tobacco and drug abuse and HIV transmission, most of the school-based programs are now touching on the dangers of tobacco. Clear messages on the health hazards of smoking are not being adequately given within the school environment [18].

A government regulation, Chapter 5: 06 of the Statute Law of Zimbabwe, prohibits the sale of alcoholic beverages or tobacco products to persons below the age of 18. Most of the shopkeepers are well aware of the age restriction, but due to the need for increased sales, they do not adhere to the requirements [19]. Because of lack of

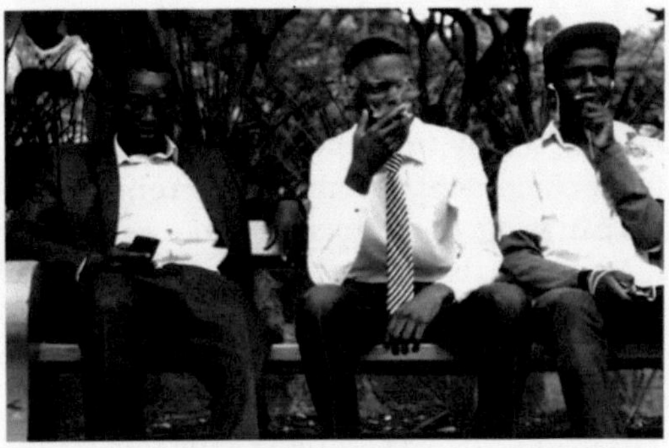

Figure 10.
Public smoking in the park [1].

enforcement of this law, the practice is further worsened because the shopkeepers know that nobody will prosecute them. Public smoking is a criminal offense under the Section 81 of Forestry Act, but no smoker has been prosecuted under the Act.

The Ministry of Health and Child Care has been using legislations such as the Public Health Act Chapter 15: 09 of 1996 and the Statutory Instrument 264 of 2002 on smoking regulations, which stipulate that smoking in public places such as halls, public offices, buses, airlines, schools, and commuter omnibuses is prohibited, to fight the scourge of public smoking. Besides drafting such policies, their enforcement and public awareness need to be considered.

9. Putting into perspective the smoking impacts

The review showed that there is substantial burden of experimental smoking among adolescents. It was established that experimentation with danger is crucial to the adolescent experience, and they start this as an act of rebellion or as a sign of maturity, but it ends up being an addictive behavior later in life. Consistent with other studies, the prevalence of smoking was higher among males, and the gap between males and females seemed not to be narrowing as previous studies intimated. This difference in prevalence between genders might be due to social and cultural acceptance of smoking among males rather than females in the country.

The low prevalence rate among the African origin group could be explained by the economic situation in Zimbabwe which has left people without any disposable income, especially those from high-density areas. The issue of increase in the prevalence of smoking across age groups might be explained by the addictive nature of the habit, and therefore students fail to stop and experience withdrawal symptoms during times of abstinence; therefore they continue smoking up to adulthood. It therefore follows that a program that successfully reduces youth smoking is likely to yield a good long-term public health benefit as most of these people who become smokers in adulthood start while they are still in their youth.

Issues related to planting alternative crops and reducing environmental and health damage from tobacco growing are contentious and complex, and any proposed solutions are likely to pose challenges for the country. The country is officially deliberating on what needs to be undertaken on coming up with alternative crops to tobacco. In country the use of taxation has been embarked on as a form of tobacco control by the Ministry of Finance and Ministry of Health. Similar efforts could be made by environmental and health authorities, who already collaborate on shared concerns such as air pollution by introducing relevant penalties.

10. Way forward in tobacco smoking control

Establishing extended producer responsibility and product stewardship programs would contribute to public health outcomes such as reducing tobacco use and increasing the cost of tobacco products, enacting new tobacco product regulations and labeling to make the product less marketable, and strengthening existing anti-litter and outdoor smoking bans. This could also include huge campaigns to raise public awareness on the environmental effects of tobacco waste, building momentum for advocacy against their irresponsible disposal. Thus numerous criteria can be used to determine how tobacco product waste should adhere to extended producer responsibility and product stewardship principles and standards [14].

Although assisting young people to avoid smoking is a widely endorsed goal of public health already, no adequate action has been taken to develop interventions that stop or reduce this habit and to make informed decisions in the country. Since the findings are almost similar to those found in Western countries, high cigarette prices and laws against youth access or adolescent tobacco education can be recommended as interventional strategies which work.

Furthermore, if health policy makers need to reduce the impact of tobacco-related diseases like tuberculosis, strategies for controlling tobacco use should be implemented now. Future studies should be implemented to monitor and evaluate the impact of the interventions.

Zimbabwe's current economic hardship, its robust tobacco growing and distribution infrastructure, and continued world demand for tobacco suggest that the government will continue to prioritize tobacco production in the absence of incentives to do otherwise. There is need to have programs that highlight the dangers of smoking. Introduction of new tobacco control and prevention programs in the country will save lives, reduce illnesses, and help reduce the economic burden associated with tobacco-related illness and lost productivity. According to available literature, non-smokers incur direct costs through passive smoking, where it has an impact on the non-smoker's health and has greater risk on property damage by fires. The financial costs are incurred by individuals who are not exposed to smoke, which include public or private healthcare costs that are tobacco related. Smoking also inflicts caring externalities that include emotional suffering experienced by non-smokers caused by the illness inflicted or death of the smoker. An increase in excise tax and the enforcement of tobacco control events would jointly reduce the cigarette demand effectively. The world is turning into a smoking epidemic, and this can be averted with the aid of these initiatives at both global and national scales.

11. Conclusion

The review exposed a plethora of adverse impacts of smoking on the country. These range from environmental degradation through deforestation and unintended veldt fires, as well as air pollution through environmental tobacco smoke. Various diseases in humans are attributed to nicotine from cigarette smoking with cancer having been identified as the most killer disease in this developing country. Leaching of chemicals from cigarette butts has also been indicated to cause extensive water pollution. Tobacco smoking tendency could not be deterred by imposition of an excise tax of 40% on cigarette sales for this tobacco-growing nation, where tobacco is in some circles viewed a major export that heavily contributes toward the economy. It is this contradictory situation that the authorities find themselves in, which compromises the legislative enforcement of various laws which are meant to reduce smoking prevalence. There is still an opportunity to mitigate the impact of smoking in the country by introducing anti-smoking health campaign programs in schools and other tertiary institutions to stop smoking tendencies in children at an early age. Excise duty could also be increased up to 75% to have a positive deterrent effect and reduce the unnecessary burden of smoking-related disease treatment on the economic budget.

Acknowledgements

We would like to thank the Zimbabwe Tobacco Board (ZTB) for making the production information which we required readily available during the process of this study. Also acknowledgments go to Zimbabwe National Statistics Agency (ZIMSTAT) for production and cigarette excise duty revenue trends. Also, we do really appreciate the solicited guidance offered by colleagues we work with at the University of Zimbabwe.

Author details

Ignatio Madanhire[1*] and Charles Mbohwa[2]

1 University of Zimbabwe, Harare, Zimbabwe

2 University of Johannesburg, Johannesburg, South Africa

*Address all correspondence to: imadanhire@gmail.com

References

[1] Bandason T, Rusakaniko S. Prevalence and associated factors of smoking among secondary school students in Harare Zimbabwe. Tobacco Induced Diseases. 2010;**8**:12. DOI: 10.1186/1617-9625-8-12

[2] van Walbeek C. Recent trends in prevalence in South Africa, some evidence from AMPS data. South African Medical Journal. 2002;**2002**(92):468-472

[3] Lown EA, Patricia A, McDaniel PA, Malone RE. Tobacco is "our industry and we must support it": Exploring the potential implications of Zimbabwe's accession to the framework convention on tobacco control. Globalization and Health. 2016;**12**:2. DOI: 10.1186/s12992-015-0139-3

[4] McDaniel PA, Intinarelli G, Malone RE. Tobacco industry issues management organizations: Creating a global corporate network to undermine public health. Globalization and Health. 2008;**4**:2. DOI: 10.1186/1744-8603-4-2

[5] Tumwine J. Implementation of the framework convention on tobacco control in Africa: Current status of legislation. International Journal of Environmental Research and Public Health. 2011;**8**(11):4312-4331. DOI: 10.3390/ijerph8114312

[6] Geist HJ. Global assessment of deforestation related to tobacco farming. Journal of Tobacco Control. 1999;**8**(1):18-28

[7] Mokdad AH, Marks JS, Stroup DF, Gerberding JL. Actual causes of death in the United States. JAMA: The Journal of the American Medical Association. 2004;**291**(10):1238-1245

[8] Machingura G. Partnering Chinese, Zimbabwe tobacco farmers embark on road to success. Available from: http://news.xinhuanet.com/english/2016-07/10/c_135502309.htm. 10 July 2016. Xinhua

[9] Xinhua C. Zimbabwe tobacco output to tumble after devastating drought. 2016. Available from: http://news.xinhuanet.com/english/2016-03/30/c_135237847.htm

[10] CCOSH. Environmental tobacco smoke (ETS): General information and health effects, Canadian: Centre for Occupational Health and Safety; 2018

[11] Dube E. Improving disaster risk reduction capacity of district civil protection units in managing veld fires: A case of Mangwe District in Matabeleland South Province, Zimbabwe. Jàmbá: Journal of Disaster Risk Studies. 2015;**7**(1), Art. #143, 13 pages

[12] Forsyth G, Kruger F, Le Maitre D. National veld fire risk assessment: Analysis of exposure of social, economic and environmental assets to veld fire hazards in South Africa, CSIR: Stellenbosch; 2010

[13] Curtis C, Collins S, Cunningham S, Stigler P, Novotny TE. Extended producer responsibility and product stewardship for tobacco product waste. International Journal of Waste Resources. 2014;**4**(3):112-133

[14] Moerman JW, Potts GE. Analysis of metals leached from smoked cigarette litter. Tobacco Control. 2017;**20** (Suppl 1):i30-i35

[15] Loker WM. The rise and fall of flue-cured tobacco in the Cop'an valley and its environmental and social consequences. Human Ecology. 2005;**33**(3):299-327

[16] The health consequences of smoking—50 years of progress: A Report of the Surgeon General,

Technical Report. US Department of Health and Human Services: Atlanta, GA; 2014

[17] Almeida G. Diversification strategies for tobacco farmers: Lessons from Brazil. In: Tobacco Control and Tobacco Farming. London: Anthem Press; 2014. pp. 211-245

[18] Gallus S, Schiaffino A, La Vecchia C, Nguyen S. Price and cigarette consumption in Europe. Tobacco Control. 2006;**15**:114-119

[19] Nelson JP. Cigarette demand, structural change, and advertising bans: International evidence, 1970–1995. Contributions to Economic Analysis & Policy. 2003;**2**:1-27

Chapter 2

What is e-Cigarette and Associated Health Risks

Narendra Maddu

Abstract

Tobacco is consumed in two forms named as smoking and smokeless tobacco. The electronic cigarettes are under the form of smoking tobacco. The electronic cigarettes (e-cigarettes) exposure has increased in recent years to the market. Many e-cigarettes contain nicotine, the primary most addictive agent in all tobacco products. We investigated the relationship between e-cigarettes and human health risks. These products may deliver sufficient nicotine for physiological responses and affects the all organs and tissues like nervous, cardiovascular, and pulmonary systems by exhibiting the effects of cytotoxic, decrease in heart rate, and extensive pulmonary damage. The e-cigarettes cannot be regarded as safe even though they are less harmful.

Keywords: electronic cigarettes, human health risks, smoking tobacco, e-cigarettes, nicotine

1. Introduction

The concept of the electronic cigarettes (EC) is quite old. It is developed in 1963 by Herbert Gilbert with a license under the name of smokeless non-tobacco cigarette. The device was first commercialized in China under the auspices of the Golden Dragon holdings. The technology of vaporization through a heating resistance was developed in 2009, and commercialized as an (ENDS) electronic nicotine delivery system [1]. EC also known as e-cigarettes, have become a popular alternative to cigarettes. The appearance of vaporized nicotine products widely referred to as electronic cigarettes or e-cigarettes (EC) has provided consumers with an alternative means of nicotine intake [2]. Information in this book has been taken from representatives of the Ministry of Health's or other regulatory body's verifications in the respective countries. There are 83 countries that have national/federal laws regulating e-cigarettes including laws related to the sale, age, advertisement, promotion, sponsorship, packaging with concern to health warning labeling and trademark, product regulation corresponding to nicotine concentration, safety, ingredients and flavors reporting taxation, use types and its toxicological evidences of e-cigarettes. Nicotine is not a carcinogenic agent, but it is a powerfully addictive substance.

The modern e-cigarette was invented in 2003 by Chinese pharmacist Hon Lik and as of 2018 most e-cigarettes are made in China [3]. Since they were first sold in 2004 their global use has risen exponentially [4]. In the United States and the United Kingdom their use is widespread. Reasons for using e-cigarettes involve trying to quit smoking, reduce risk, or save money, though some use them recreationally [5]. There are around 500 brands of e-cigarettes, with global sales in excess of US $ 7 billion [6].

2. What is e-cigarette?

The appearance of vaporized nicotine products widely referred to as e-cigarettes (EC) has provided consumers with an alternative means of nicotine intake [2]. An electronic cigarette or e-cigarette is also known as e-cigs, electronic nicotine delivery systems (ENDS) or electronic non-nicotine delivery systems (ENNDS), electronic smoking devices (ESDs), personal vaporizers (PVs), is a handheld electronic device that simulates the feeling of smoking. It works by heating a liquid to generate an aerosol, commonly called a "vapor", that the user inhales [4]. Using e-cigarettes is commonly referred to as vaping. The liquid in the e-cigarette, called e-liquid, or e-juice, is usually made of nicotine, propylene glycol, glycerine, and flavorings. Not all e-liquids contain nicotine. Most e-cigarettes contain a liquid, known as e-liquid or e-juice that contains a mixture of the following:

Water

Propylene glycol (PG)

Vegetable glycerin (VG)

Flavouring

Nicotine.

Different strengths of nicotine are available. The best way to assess the strength is by looking at the concentration which is expressed as milligrams of nicotine per millilitre of liquid (mg/ml), or a percentage (**Table 1**).

S. no	Strength	mg/ml	Percentage (%)
1	Nicotine free	0.0	0
2	Low	8.0	0.8
3	Medium	12.0	1.2
4	High	24.0	2.4
5	Highest	36.0	3.6

Table 1.
Different concentration/percentage of e-cigarettes.

3. Construction of e-cigars

An electronic cigarette is a battery-powered vaporizer [7]. The primary parts that make up an e-cigarette are a mouthpiece, a cartridge, a heating element/atomizer, a microprocessor, a battery, and possibly a LED light on the end. An atomizer comprises a small heating element that vaporizes e-liquid and wicking material that draws liquid onto the coil. When the user pushes a button, or (in some variations) activates a pressure sensor by inhaling, the heating element then atomizes the liquid solution. The e-liquid reaches a temperature of roughly 100–250°C (212–482°F) within a chamber to create an aerosolized vapor. The user inhales the aerosol, commonly called vapor, rather than cigarette smoke. The aerosol provides a flavor and feels similar to tobacco smoking. There are three main types of e-cigarettes:

1. cigalikes, looking like cigarettes;

2. eGos, bigger than cigalikes with refillable liquid tanks and;

3. mods, assembled with basic parts or by altering existing products.

First generation e-cigarettes tend to look like tobacco cigarettes and so are called "cigalikes" [8]. Most cigalikes look like cigarettes but there is some variation in size. Second generation devices are larger overall and look less like tobacco cigarettes. Third generation devices include mechanical mods and variable voltage devices. The fourth generation includes sub ohm tanks and temperature control devices. The power source is the biggest component of an e-cigarette, which is frequently a rechargeable lithium-ion battery [3] (**Figures 1** and **2**).

The majority of toxic chemicals found in tobacco smoke are absent in e-cigarette aerosol [9]. Those present are mostly below 1% of the corresponding levels in tobacco smoke. e-Cigarettes create an aerosol that can contain toxicants and traces

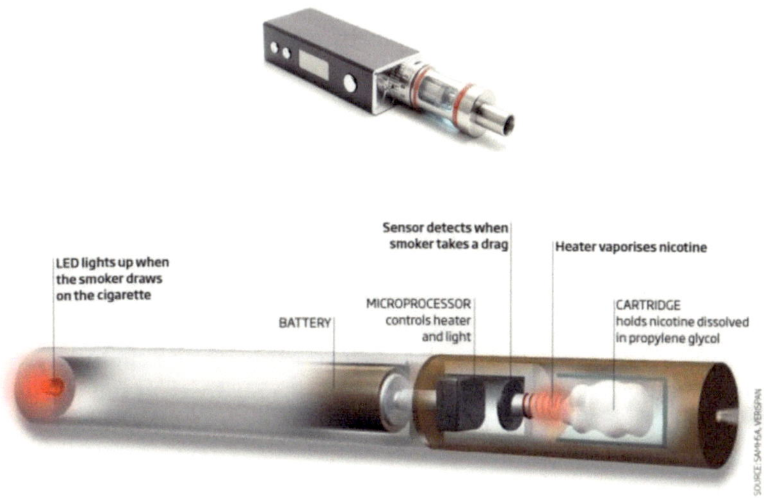

Figure 1.
Structure of e-cigar.

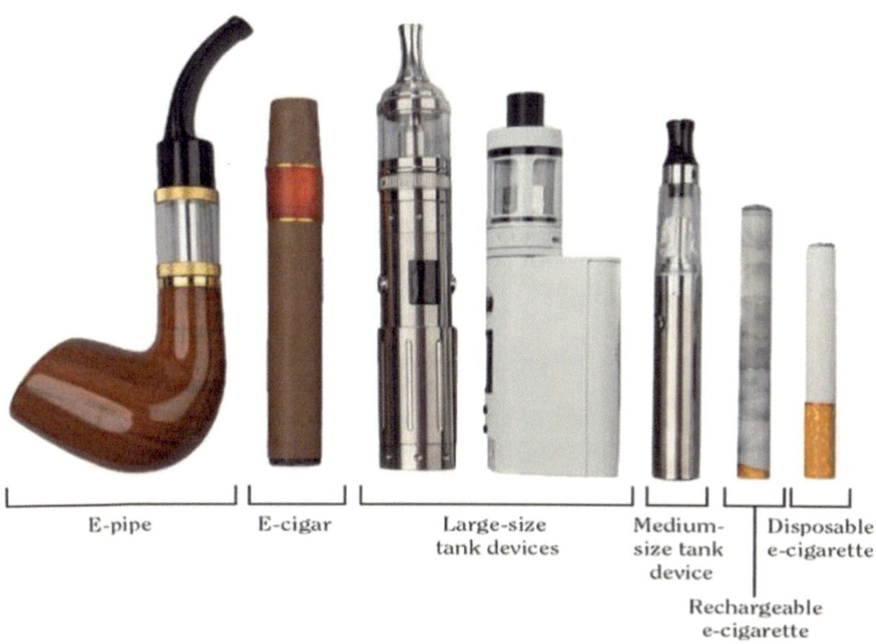

Figure 2.
Types of e-cigs.

of heavy metals at levels permissible in inhalation medicines [4] and potentially harmful chemicals not found in tobacco smoke at concentrations permissible by workplace safety standards.

4. Content of e-liquid

The liquid is composed of carrier solvents in e-cigarette, such as glycerol and/or propylene glycol. Aerosol generated from an e-cigarette is commonly but inaccurately referred to as 'vapour'. Vapour refers to the gaseous state of a substance; in contrast, an aerosol is a suspension of fine particles of liquid, solid or both in a gas form. Both the particulate and gases phase are mixtures of chemical substances in e-cigarette aerosols. The e-cigarette aerosol simulates cigarette smoke [10]. A puff of the aerosol is delivered into the user's mouth and lungs through inhalation, after which the remaining aerosol is exhaled into the environment [11]. These products are commercialised in various forms or 'models' with different design characteristics and generate different physical and chemical characteristics during operation.

e-cigarettes are becoming ever more popular, a concerning trend given limited information about their research. Marketers of e-cigarettes have made a variety of claims indicating that e-cigarettes are safer than conventional cigarettes and that their use facilitates smoking cessation [12]. However, e-cigarette manufacturers do not provide complete information on the chemicals used in the manufacturing process or the chemicals that may be released or synthesized during the aerosol generation process that occurs during use. Minimal valid research data are available on e-cigarette emissions. Furthermore, nicotine levels are intentionally formulated to create target strengths, yet measured levels may not match the label claim [13]. Consequently, safety concerns exist regarding e-cigarette user exposure to harmful and potentially harmful constituents (HPHCs), including nicotine, which has the potential to cause addiction and other adverse events [14].

5. Harmful chemicals in electronic cigarettes

While a limited numbers of studies have been conducted on EC to date, scientific studies have been identified hundreds of chemicals in the vapors of EC. About 42 chemicals are identified in the ECs, among which main stream smoke exposure can be especially harmful to health and some are emitted in the second hand smoke. They are listed in **Table 2**.

Main stream smoke	Second hand smoke
Acetaldehyde and acetone	Benzene
Acrolein	Farmaldehyde and benzaldehyde
Cadmium, nickle and lead	Diethylene glycol
Chromium	Nicotine and N-nitrosonornicotine
Phenol and propylene glycol	
O-methylbenzaldehyde	

Table 2.
Chemicals in e-cigarettes.

6. Frequency of e-cig users in global world

When the FDA commissioned their 2018 report on ENDS which they label as a Tobacco Product, the authors chose to use the term e-cigarettes for some use e-juice without nicotine [15]. At least 52% of smokers or ex-smokers in one area have vaped [16]. In the US, as of 2014, 12.6% of adults had used an e-cigarette at least once and approximately 3.7% were still using them [6], 1.1% of adults were daily users. Non-smokers and former smokers who had quit more than 4 years earlier were extremely unlikely to be current users [17]. In the UK, there were about 2.6 million users in 2015 which is about 18% of current smokers and about 5% of the population. About 59% of current smokers said they had tried them. In France in 2014, between 7.7 and 9.2 million people have tried e-cigarettes and 1.1–1.9 million use them on a daily basis. About 67% of French smokers use e-cigarettes to reduce or quit smoking. French people who have tried e-cigarettes, 9% have never smoked tobacco. Of the 1.2% who had recently stopped tobacco smoking at the time of the survey, 84% credited e-cigarettes as essential in quitting.

Although smoking among young people has declined over the last 5 years, this has coincided with a growth in the use of alternative nicotine products [18]. Some young people who have tried an e-cigarette have never smoked tobacco, so vaping can be a starting point for nicotine use [19]. The evidence on whether e-cigarettes are a gateway to tobacco smoking in later life is mixed and contradictory. e-Cigarettes, also known as vape pens, cartridges and pens, differ from traditional marijuana cigarettes in several respects. e-Cigarettes may be used with other substances and cartridges can potentially be filled with e-liquid containing substances other than nicotine, thus serving as a new way to deliver other psychoactive drugs, for example THC [20].

The amount of nicotine found in 13 inhalations from an e-cigarette with fluid containing 18 mg/ml nicotine was estimated to be equivalent to the amount found in a typical tobacco cigarette containing 0.5 mg nicotine [21]. Most medical organizations, including international organizations such as the WHO and those in the US, feel there is insufficient evidence to routinely recommend electronic cigarettes for use in smoking cessation [4] other medical organizations, particularly British ones, state e-cigarettes are a reasonable third-best alternative for smokers who are unable to quit. The available research on e-cigarette use for smoking cessation is limited. Some medical authorities recommend that e-cigarettes have a role in smoking cessation, and others disagree.

A 2016 meta-analysis based on 20 different studies found that smokers who vaped were 28% less likely to quit than those who had not tried electronic cigarettes. In the US, e-cigarettes have not been subject to the same efficacy testing as nicotine replacement products. Several authorities, including the World Health Organization, feel there is not enough evidence to recommend e-cigarettes for quitting smoking, and there are studies showing a decline in smoking cessation among dual users [22, 23]. Nicotine-containing e-cigarettes were associated with greater effectiveness for quitting smoking than e-cigarettes without nicotine. e-Cigarettes without nicotine may reduce tobacco cravings because of the smoking-related physical stimuli.

7. Adverse effects of vaping

The health risks of e-cigarettes are uncertain. Their long-term health effects are not known. When used by non-smokers, e-cigarettes can lead to nicotine addiction, and there is concern that children could start smoking after using e-cigarettes. So far, no serious adverse effects have been reported in trials. Less serious adverse effects include throat and mouth irritation, vomiting, nausea, and coughing.

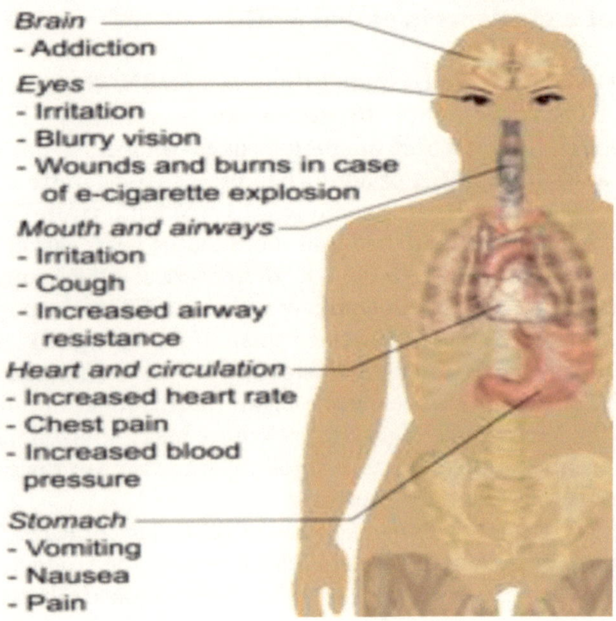

Figure 3.
Adverse effects of vaping on human health.

The European Commission recently concluded that the use of refillable electronic e-cigarettes, and the potential exposure to e-liquids containing nicotine in high strength, may pose harm to public health. It is found to exert adverse effects on lung and brain development in addition to the other parts. Nicotine can also have a little effect on human haemodynamics [19] (**Figure 3**).

Compared to conventional cigarettes, similar substances with potential carcinogenic or toxic effects are found in aerosol from electronic cigarettes, but in lower concentrations, whereas emitted reactive oxygen radicals appear comparable [24]. Although males more commonly reported any type of tobacco use as well as e-cigs, 9.5% of American high-school females reported current use of e-cigs, carrying a significant risk of using e-cigs in future pregnancies [25]. Although research is emerging around e-cigs in general, there continues to be a lack of scientific evidence regarding the safety and risks of e-cig use on maternal and fetal health, even though adverse health effects of nicotine on maternal and fetal outcomes are documented e-cigarettes, often touted as a safer alternative to cigarette smoking, may modify the DNA in the oral cells of users, potentially increasing the risk of cancer. Health risks conferred by smoking ordinary tobacco cigarettes include a number of non-communicable diseases, such as chronic obstructive pulmonary disease (COPD), lung cancer and cardiovascular diseases (**Figure 4**).

The long-term effects of e-cigarette use are unknown. Improvements in lung function and pulmonary health have been demonstrated among smokers who have switched to e-cigarettes [26]. WHO [4] reported that ENDS use poses serious threats to adolescents and fetuses. It is also thought that nicotine can create an increased risk of sudden infant death syndrome (SIDS). Other adverse outcomes include disruptive behavioral disorders, attention deficit hyperactivity disorder, reduced respiratory compliance, forced expiratory flow, and impaired lung function. It is also thought that electronic cigarette use can expose individuals to oxidants. Some studies have associated electronic cigarette use with an increased oxidative stress [27]. Aside from toxicity, there are also risks from misuse or accidents such as contact with liquid nicotine [28] (**Figure 5**).

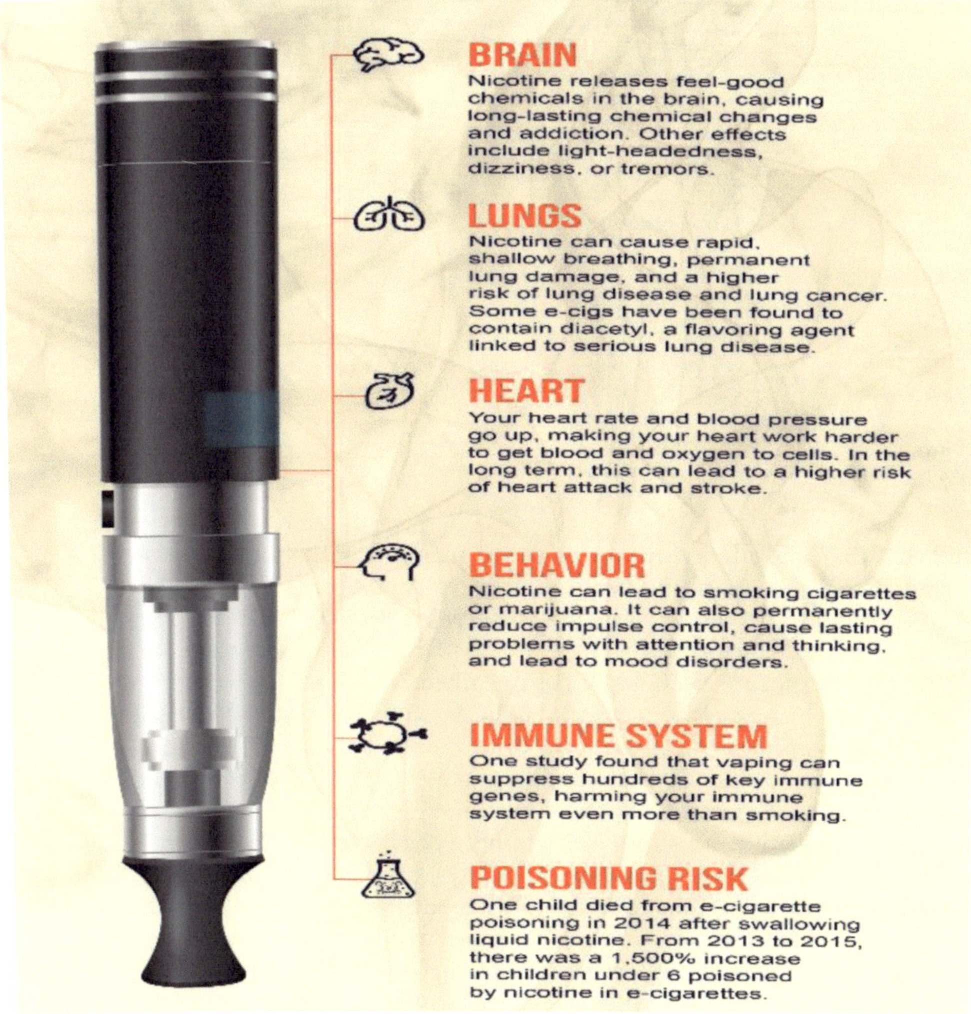

Figure 4.
E-cigs—effect on the body parts.

e-Cigarette users who use e-cigarettes that contain nicotine are exposed to its potentially harmful effects [29]. Nicotine is associated with cardiovascular disease, potential birth defects, and poisoning. The vapor has been found to contain flavors, propylene glycol, glycerin, nicotine, tiny amounts of toxicants, carcinogens, heavy metals, and metal nanoparticles, and other harmful chemicals [19]. There is limited information available on the environmental issues around production, use, and disposal of e-cigarettes that use cartridges. Regulatory limits should be contemplated for levels of some of the more worrisome chemicals as well as for total flavor chemical levels.

Human and animal studies have found that nicotine exposure from e-cigarettes during adolescence adversely affects cognitive development [30], and animal research suggests that it has more severe impacts on the most vulnerable parts of the brain. One such region adversely affected by nicotine within the adolescent brain is the limbic system, which modulates drug reward, cognition, and emotion [31]. Nicotine is poisonous, and e-cigarette use or misuse can lead to nicotine poisoning via ingestion, inhalation, or absorption of nicotine via the skin or eyes. Early signs of accidental nicotine exposure include quickened tachycardia, diaphoresis, nausea,

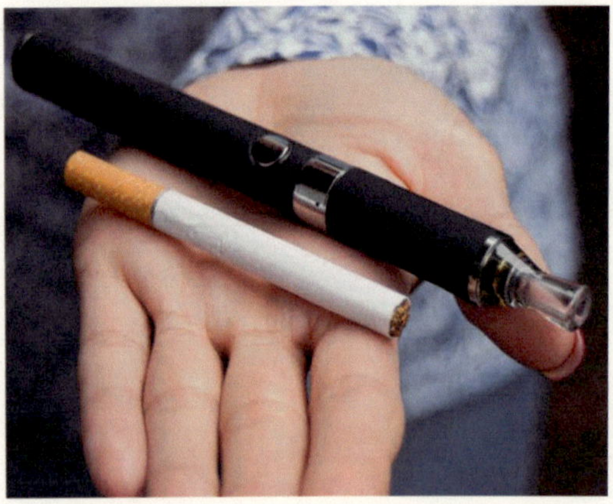

Figure 5.
Swithing to e-cigarettes—not a healthy choice.

and vomiting, late effects include hypotension, hypoventilation and other effects include coma, seizure, respiratory, cardiac arrest and death.

As the usage of e-cigarettes increased between 2012 and 2015, the accidental nicotine exposure rate increased by 1398.2% in the US [32]. The absolute impact from passive exposure to EC vapor has the potential to lead to adverse health effects. The risk from being passively exposed to EC vapor is likely to be less than the risk from passive exposure to conventional cigarette smoke. Nicotine in tobacco smoke is absorbed into the bloodstream rapidly, and e-cigarette vapor is relatively slow in this regard [8]. e-Cigarettes have been advanced as a strategy to reduce the addictive levels of nicotine in cigarettes. Nicotine, a key ingredient in most e-liquids, is a highly addictive substance. Nicotine stimulates regions of the cortex associated with reward, pleasure and reducing anxiety. When nicotine intake stops, withdrawal symptoms include cravings for nicotine, anger/irritability, anxiety, depression, impatience, trouble sleeping, restlessness, hunger or weight gain, and difficulty concentrating. During pregnancy, the nicotine exposure increases the risk for eclampsia, premature birth, still birth, reduced birth weight, reduced lung function at birth, apnea, cleft lip and palate and probably effects muscle and skeletal development in the new-born child [33]. The nicotine content in e-cigarettes is adequate to cause or sustain nicotine dependence.

Systems toxicology investigations indicated that nicotine exposure also affected metabolic pathways the in liver, including upregulation of fatty acid beta-oxidation, cholesterol synthesis, gluconeogenesis, and ketone body formation pathways. Both standard and systems toxicology endpoints demonstrated very limited biological effects of propyleneglycol (PG), and vegetable glycerin (VG) aerosol with no signs of toxicity. Systems toxicology analyses detected biological effects of nicotine exposure, which included up-regulation of the xenobiotic-metabolizing enzymes CYP1A1 and FMO3 in the lung and metabolic effects, likely interlinked with a generalized stress response to nicotine present in the exposure aerosols [34].

Because e-cigarettes are relatively new to the scene, yet a very little research is available about how they impact the body. Still, numerous studies already offer crucial insights about how vaping might affect both your risk of type two diabetes and your management of the disease. However, the safety of e-cigarettes is debated, and a growing body of evidence is suggesting several adverse health effects. It's well known that traditional cigarettes can increase the risk of type two diabetes and related complications, but researchers are still analyzing the potential relationship between e-cigarettes and the disease.

e-Cigarette use is associated with a 42% increased risk of myocardial infarction, or heart attack, for which people with diabetes already have a heightened risk. Smoking e-cigarettes can lead to the mobilization of cells called endothelial progenitor cells (EPCs) to damaged blood vessels, a reaction that also occurs after people smoke traditional cigarettes. Over time, repeated and chronic mobilization of EPCs can actually deplete them. Lower levels of EPCs are also associated with both cardiovascular disease and type two diabetes. The nicotine in e-cigarettes could also affect blood sugar followed by hemoglobin A1C to rise by 34% that indicate a higher risk of complications from diabetes, including eye disease, heart disease, and kidney disease [35].

Nicotine and cigarette smoking is known to promote weight loss and suppress appetite. Since becoming available in 2007, the use of electronic cigarettes (e-cig) has increased dramatically in the US, however there are still very few studies that examine the long-term consequences of e-vapor, particularly in the context of appetite regulation or weight management [36]. The marketing of e-cigarette use as a safer alternative to cigarette smoking has led to an increasing use even in pregnancy. The nicotine consumed by e-cigarettes is similar to that consumed by cigarette smoking. Animal studies confirm the dangers of nicotine to the developing fetus. More research needs to be done specifically assessing e-cigarette use, pregnancy, and pregnancy outcomes [37].

In vitro studies have shown that cytotoxic effects vary among EC refill fluids. A few flavored chemicals (such as cinnamaldehyde) have toxicity at the concentrations used in EC [38], and stem cells are more sensitive than differentiated adult lung cells to EC products [39]. Recent studies have further shown that EC aerosols induced DNA strand breaks and reduced cell survival *in vitro* [40]. EC aerosols also reduced endothelial barrier function in cultured lung microvascular endothelial cells and increased inflammation and oxidative stress in mice [41]. Most case reports show that the health of children and adults can be negatively affected by EC products and that if death does not occur, negative effects can be reversed. Data further indicate that EC use can cause negative health effects in previously healthy individuals and exacerbate pre-existing conditions [42]. Research will help make electronic cigarettes more effective as smoking substitutes and will better define and further reduce residual risks from use to as low as possible, by establishing appropriate quality control and standards.

Mayer [43] suggested that the acute dose associated with a lethal outcome would be 500–1000 mg. Taking into account that voluminous vomiting is the first and characteristic symptom of nicotine ingestion, it seems that far higher levels of nicotine need to be ingested in order to have lethal consequences. However, due to the paucity of experimental data and contradictory evidence, it is difficult to draw conclusive outcomes regarding toxicological, immunological and clinical impacts of e-cig aerosols. Excessive vaping has been reported to induce inflammatory responses including mitogen-activated protein kinase, Janus tyrosine kinase/signal transducer and activator of transcription and nuclear factor-κB signaling, similar to that induced by tobacco smoke. Based on recent evidence, prolonged exposure to some constituents of e-cig aerosols might result in respiratory complications such as asthma, chronic obstructive pulmonary disease and inflammation.

A study using young healthy human airway epithelial cells showed that e-cigarette fluid promotes pro-inflammatory cytokine IL-6 production and human rhinovirus infection. Human lung fibroblasts exposed to e-cigarette liquid showed cell stress and other phenotypic abnormalities. A study in human embryonic stem cells also showed dysregulation of gene expression indicating a negative effect of e-cigarette use on heart development. Some studies found that at biologically relevant doses, vaporized e-liquids induced increased DNA strand breaks and cell death, and decreased

Chemical constituents	Permissible limit	Toxic effect	Molecular mechanism of toxicity	Reference
Acetaldehyde	45–270 ppm for 1 h	Eye, skin and respiratory tract irritation on acute exposure; pulmonary oedema and necrosis on higher exposures [46, 47]	Readily binds to protein and DNA, forming damaging adducts and impairing normal function and enzyme activity	[48, 49]
Acetone	750–1000 ppm per 8 h	Respiratory irritant in small quantities; CNS depression and cardiorespiratory failure in large amounts [50, 51]	Metabolism in high amounts is not possible, leading to its accumulation and toxicity	[50]
Acrolein	0.1 ppm per 8 h	Highly toxic respiratory and cardiovascular toxicant [51, 52]	Highly reactive, leading to DNA and protein adduction, endoplasmic reticulum stress, membrane damage, mitochondrial disruption, oxidative stress and immune dysfunction	[53]
Cadmium	5 μg m^{-3} of air for 8 h	Pulmonary changes with obstructive damage, renal dysfunction and teratogenicity in animals [54]	Interacts with DNA repair machinery, acts as a catalyst for ROS production, increases lipid peroxidation and induces apoptosis in cellular systems	[55, 56]
Chromium	0.5 mg m^{-3}	Nasal ulcers and perforations, lung and prostate cancers [57]	Under physiological conditions, can produce reactive intermediates, hydrogen peroxide and GSH, which can attack DNA, protein and membrane lipids	[58]
Formaldehyde	0.3 ng m^{-3}	Respiratory inflammation, pneumonia and bronchitis, neurological symptoms [57]	Highly reactive electrophilic reagent that can easily attach to neutrophilic biological targets, leading to formation of harmful adducts and ROS	[59]
Nicotine	0.5 mg m^{-3}	Hypertension, tachycardia, vasoconstriction, bronchorrhea, hyperpnoea [60, 61]	Toxicity attributed to oxidative damage, lipid peroxidation and DNA adduct formation	[62]
N-Nitrosamine	0.3 ng m^{-3}	Carcinogen [57]	Forms diazonium or oxynium ions which cause alkylating DNA	[63]
Toluene	200 ppm per 8 h	Neurotoxicity including euphoria, depression, cognitive impairment [64]	Metabolises to form hippurate ions resulting in metabolic acidosis and hypokalaemia	[65]
Lead	50 μg m^{-3} per 8 h	Neurotoxin, cardiotoxin, behavioral and developmental changes [66]	Causes oxidative stress and ionic imbalance	[67]

CNS, central nervous system; ROS, reactive oxygen species; GSH, glutathione.

Table 3.
Chemical constituents of e-cigarettes and its molecular mechanism(s) of toxicity.

clonogenic survival in both normal epithelial and head and neck squamous cell carcinoma cell lines independently of nicotine content [40]. Exposure to e-cigarette vapour also decreased the expression of cardiac transcription factors in cardiac progenitor cells, suggesting a persistent delay in differentiation [44].

Canistro et al. [45] found that e-cigs have a powerful booster effect on phase-I carcinogen-bioactivating enzymes, including activators of polycyclic aromatic hydrocarbons (PAHs), and increase oxygen free radical production and DNA oxidation to 8-hydroxy2'-deoxyguanosine. Furthermore, we found that e-cigs damage DNA not only at chromosomal level in peripheral blood, such as strand breaks in leucocytes and micronuclei formation in reticulocytes, but also at gene level such as point mutations in urine. Despite its short comings, the work presented here strongly raises the possibility that e-cig consumption under certain conditions leads to toxicological outcomes directly and indirectly damaging DNA in the rat.

After e-cig aerosol exposure, the overall lipid composition of rat plasma was markedly affected with significant increases in the content of esterified cholesterol, total cholesterol and triglycerides. Also observed a significant increase in cytochrome P450 (CYP)-CYP1A1/2, CYP2B1/2 and CYP3A to an enhanced cancer risk from the widely bioactivated e-cig vapour procarcinogens associated with an increased risk of lung cancer with CYP induction and/or CYP polymorphisms (**Table 3**).

Three categories of negative health effects were identified: systemic effects, nicotine poisoning, and mechanical injury. Systemic effects include respiratory, gastrointestinal, cardiovascular, immunological and neurological systems. Patients with negative effects were experiencing symptoms such as shortness of breath and cough. For the individuals with bronchiolitis, acute eosinophilic pneumonia, and pneumonia with bilateral pleural effusions, the onset of adverse health effects occurred within 3–7 days of EC use. Dyspnea, productive cough, mild tachycardia, exogenous lipoid pneumonia. Bronchial syndrome associated with deterioration of pulmonary function test, sub-acute bronchial toxicity, pleuritic chest pain [68]. Relapsed medically refractive ulcerative colitis, abdominal distention, respiratory distress, isolated chronic necrotizing enterocolitis. Asymptomatic acute and paroxysmal atrial fibrillation (AF). Acute myocardial infarction. Reversible cerebral vasoconstriction syndrome. Nicotine poisoning effects involves accidental poisoning, poisoning caused by intentional abuse or misuse and suicidal attempts which are symptomized by sudden onset vomiting, irritability, tachycardia, flushing, salivation and nausea, dizziness, mild tremor, shivering, cardiovascular resuscitation and full body seizures, multiple acute infarcts severe anoxic brain injury and death [69]. Mechanical injury caused by spontaneous explosion of EC battery. Also include oral trauma; tooth avulsion and severe mouth burns [70].

8. Harm reduction and safety

Awaiting future observations from current exposure must be taken into consideration when assessing harmful effects of e-cigarettes, and a precautionary principle is highly relevant. e-Cigarettes can reduce smokers exposure to carcinogens and other toxic substances found in tobacco, and are very likely less harmful than tobacco cigarettes [71]. This is a motivation for many e-cigarette users. The American Association of Public Health Physicians (AAPHP) suggests those who are unwilling to quit tobacco smoking or unable to quit with medical advice and pharmaceutical methods should consider other nicotine containing products such as electronic cigarettes and smokeless tobacco for long term use instead of smoking. The safety of electronic cigarettes is uncertain [22]. Tobacco smoke contains 100 known carcinogens, and 900 potentially cancer-causing chemicals, none of which has been found in more than trace quantities in e-cigarette vapor. A 2014 review recommended that regulations for e-cigarettes could be similar to those for dietary supplements or cosmetic products to not limit their potential for harm reduction [72]. A 2012 review found e-cigarettes could considerably reduce traditional cigarettes use and they likely could be used as a lower risk replacement for traditional cigarettes, but there is not enough data on their safety and efficacy to draw definite conclusions.

9. Conclusions

Electronic cigarettes may help smokers stop their smoking, and the included studies did not find any serious side effects associated with their use for short duration up to 2 years. E-cigarettes are very limited and can be puzzling, so having the basic understanding of the mechanism of action, current regulation and health effects of this product. Impact on smoking cessation is unclear. Overall, the wide variability in products and lack of standardized testing methods makes evaluation of the available data in scientific community. It will be interesting to see the turn of events that e-cigarettes has in its role with tobacco users.

Conflict of interest

The authors report no declarations of interest.

Author details

Narendra Maddu
Department of Biochemistry, Sri Krishnadevaraya University, Ananthapuramu, Andhra Pradesh, India

*Address all correspondence to: dr.narendramaddu@gmail.com

References

[1] Leduc C, Quoix E. Is there a role for e-cigarettes in smoking cessation? Therapeutic Advances in Respiratory Disease. 2016;**10**:130-135

[2] Ali I, Patthi B, Singla A, Malhi R, Niraj LK, Dhama K. Role of e-cigarettes in smoking cessation: A systematic review. Journal Indian Association Public Health Dent. 2018;**16**:94-102

[3] Oren R, Giuseppe AV, Abraham RZ. Are e-cigarettes a safe and good alternative to cigarette smoking? Annals of the New York Academy of Sciences. 2014;**1340**:65-74

[4] WHO. Electronic Nicotine Delivery Systems. Section on Tobacco Control Pediatrics. From the American Academy of Pediatrics Policy Statement. November 2015;**136**(5):1-13

[5] Rahman MA, Hann N, Wilson A, Worrall-Carter L. Electronic cigarettes: Patterns of use, health effects, use in smoking cessation and regulatory issues. Tobacco Induced Diseases. 2014;**12**:21

[6] Charlotte A, Gindi SRM. Electronic cigarette use among adults: United States, 2014. Centers for Disease Control and Prevention. 2015;**217**:1-8

[7] Pasquale C, Davide C, Gabriella P, Cristina R, Riccardo P. The emerging phenomenon of electronic cigarettes. Expert Review of Respiratory Medicine. 2012;**6**:63-74

[8] Farsalinos KE, Spyrou A, Tsimopoulou K, Stefopoulos C, Romagna G, Voudris V. Nicotine absorption from electronic cigarette use: Comparison between first and new-generation devices. Scientific Reports. 2014;**4**:4133

[9] Igor B. Peering through the mist: Systematic review of what the chemistry of contaminants in electronic cigarettes tells us about health risks. BMC Public Health. 2014;**14**:18

[10] Trtchounian A, Williams M, Talbot P. Conventional and electronic cigarettes (e-cigarettes) have different smoking characteristics. Nicotine & Tobacco Research. 2010;**2**:905-912

[11] Pauly J, Li Q, Barry MB. Tobacco-free electronic cigarettes and cigars deliver nicotine and generate concern. Tobacco Control. 2007;**16**:357

[12] Henningfield JE, Zaatari GS. Electronic nicotine delivery systems: Emerging science foundation for policy. Tobacco Control. 2010;**19**:89-90

[13] Goniewicz ML, Kuma T, Gawron M, et al. Nicotine levels in electronic cigarettes. Nicotine & Tobacco Research. 2013;**15**:158-166

[14] Chen I. FDA summary of adverse events on electronic cigarettes. Nicotine & Tobacco Research. 2013;**15**:615-616

[15] Born H, Persky M, Kraus DH, Peng R, Amin MR, Branski RC. Electronic cigarettes: A primer for clinicians. Otolaryngology and Head and Neck Surgery. 2015;**153**:5-14

[16] Alawsi F, Nour R, Prabhu S. Are e-cigarettes a gateway to smoking or a pathway to quitting? British Dental Journal. 2015;**219**:111-115

[17] Cristine DD, Daniel GP, Michael SB, Andrea VC, Jennifer P, Raymond NS, et al. Patterns of electronic cigarette use among adults in the United States. Nicotine & Tobacco Research. 2015;**18**:715-719

[18] Dana L, Risa H, Terry G, Beverly-Xaviera W, Michael W, Judith Z. The changing face of tobacco use among United States youth. Current Drug Abuse Reviews. 2014;**7**:29-43

[19] Grana R, Benowitz N, Glantz SA. E-cigarette: A scientific review. Circulation. 2014;**129**:1972-1986

[20] Christian I, Mariangela de C, Aurelie B, Vincent V, Nicolas CL, Bernard F. E-cigarettes: A review of new trends in cannabis use. International Journal of Environmental Research and Public Health. 2015;**12**:9988-10008

[21] Geiss O, Bianchi I, Barahona F, Barrero-Moreno J. Characterisation of mainstream and passive vapours emitted by selected electronic cigarettes. International Journal of Hygiene and Environmental Health. 2015;**218**:169-180

[22] Siu AL. Behavioral and pharmacotherapy interventions for tobacco smoking cessation in adults, including pregnant women: U.S. preventive services task force recommendation statement. Annals of Internal Medicine. 2015;**163**:622-634

[23] Sara K, Stanton GA. E-cigarettes and smoking cessation in real-world and clinical settings: A systematic review and meta-analysis. The Lancet Respiratory Medicine. 2016;**4**:116-128

[24] Lerner CA, Sundar IK, Watson RM. Environmental health hazards of e-cigarettes and their components: Oxidants and copper in e-cigarette aerosols. Environmental Pollution. 2015;**198**:100-107

[25] Wagner NJ, Camerota M, Propper C. Prevalence and perceptions of electronic cigarette use during pregnancy. Maternal and Child Health Journal. 2017;**21**:1655-1661

[26] Polosa R, Campagna D, Caponnetto P. What to advise to respiratory patients intending to use electronic cigarettes. Discovery Medicine. 2015;**20**:155-161

[27] Cai H, Wang C. Graphical review: The redox dark side of e-cigarettes; exposure to oxidants and public health concerns. Redox Biology. 2017;**13**:402-406

[28] Durmowicz EL. The impact of electronic cigarettes on the paediatric population. Tobacco Control. 2014;**23**:41-46

[29] Cheng T. Chemical evaluation of electronic cigarettes. Tobacco Control. 2014;**23**:11-17

[30] Lucinda EJ, Rebecca BE, Terry PF, Van TT, Tim MA. Nicotine and the developing human. American Journal of Preventive Medicine. 2015;**49**:286-293

[31] Menglu Y, Sarah C. Nicotine and the adolescent brain. Journal of Physiology. 2015;**593**:3397-3412

[32] Preethi G, Henry SA, Marcel CJ, Thitphalak C, Gary SA. E-cigarette and liquid nicotine exposures among young children. Pediatrics. 2018;**141**:e20173361

[33] Baba S, Wikstrom AK, Stephansson O, Cnattingius S. Influence of smoking and snuff cessation on risk of preterm birth. European Journal of Epidemiology. 2012;**27**:297-304

[34] Phillips B, Titz B, Kogel U, Sharma D, Leroy P, Xian Y, et al. Toxicity of the main electronic cigarette components, propylene glycol, glycerin, and nicotine, in Sprague-Dawley rats in a 90-day OECD inhalation study complemented by molecular endpoints. Food and Chemical Toxicology. 2017;**109**:315-332

[35] Antoniewicz L, Bosson JA, Kuhl J, Abdel-Halim SM, Kiessling A, Mobarrez F, et al. Electronic cigarettes increase endothelial progenitor cells in the blood of healthy volunteers. Atherosclerosis. 2016;**255**:179-185

[36] Breit M, Hoskinson H, Pitzer C, Wu Z, Bryner R, Olfert IM. Effects of electronic cigarette vapor on body mass,

food intake, and body composition. Federation of American Societies for Experimental Biology Journal. 2017;**31**:1037.6

[37] Whittington JR, Simmons PM, Phillips AM, Gammill SK, Cen R, Magann EF, et al. The use of electronic cigarettes in pregnancy: A review of the literature. Obstetrical & Gynecological Survey. 2018;**73**:544-549

[38] Behar RZ, Davis B, Wang Y, Bahl V, Lin S, Talbot P. Identification of toxicants in cinnamon-flavored electronic cigarette refill fluids. Toxicology In Vitro. 2014;**28**:198-208

[39] Bahl V, Lin S, Xu N, Davis B, Wang YH, Talbot P. Comparison of electronic cigarette refill fluid cytotoxicity using embryonic and adult models. Reproductive Toxicology. 2012;**34**:529537

[40] Yu V, Rahimy M, Korrapati A. Electronic cigarettes induce DNA strand breaks and cell death independently of nicotine in cell lines. Oral Oncology. 2016;**52**:58-65

[41] Schweitzer KS, Chen SX, Law S. Endothelial disruptive proinflammatory effects of nicotine and e-cigarette vapor exposures. American Journal of physiology Lung Cellular and Molecular Physiology. 2015;**309**:175-187

[42] Hua M, Talbot P. Potential health effects of electronic cigarettes: A systematic review of case reports. Preventive Medicine Reports. 2016;**4**:169-178

[43] Mayer B. How much nicotine kills a human? Tracing back the generally accepted lethal dose to dubious self-experiments in the nineteenth century. Archives of Toxicology. 2013;**88**:5-7

[44] Palpant NJ, Hofsteen P, Pabon L, Reinecke H, Murry CE. Cardiac development in zebrafish and human embryonic stem cells is inhibited by exposure to tobacco cigarettes and e-cigarettes. PLoS ONE. 2015;**10**:e0126259

[45] Canistro D, Vivarelli F, Cirillo S, Marquillas CB, Annamaria B, Lazzaretti M, et al. E-cigarettes induce toxicological effects that can raise the cancer risk. Scientific Reports. 2017;**7**(2028):1-9

[46] United States Environmental Protection Agency. Acetaldehyde Hazard Summary. Washington, DC: United States Environmental Protection Agency; 2000

[47] Feron VJ, Kruysse A, Woutersen RA. Respiratory tract tumours in hamsters exposed to acetaldehyde vapour alone or simultaneously to benzo(a)pyrene or diethylnitrosamine. European Journal of Cancer & Clinical Oncology. 1982;**18**:13-31

[48] Setshedi M, Wands JR, Monte SM. Acetaldehyde adducts in alcoholic liver disease. Oxidative Medicine and Cellular Longevity. 2010;**3**:178-185

[49] Lieber CS. Metabolic effects of acetaldehyde. Biochemical Society Transactions. 1988;**16**:241-247

[50] US Department of Health and Human Services, Public Health Service, Agency for Toxic Substances and Disease Registry. Toxicological Profile for Acetone. Atlanta, GA: US Department of Health and Human Services, Public Health Service; 1994

[51] Talhout R, Schulz T, Florek E, et al. Hazardous compounds in tobacco smoke. International Journal of Environmental Research and Public Health. 2011;**8**:613-628

[52] Agency for Toxic Substances and Disease Registry. Medical Management Guidelines for Acrolein. Available from: www.atsdr.cdc.gov/MMG/MMG.

asp?id=552&tid=102 [Accessed: 11 June 2017. Date last updated: 21 Octomber 2014]

[53] Moghe A, Ghare S, Lamoreau B, et al. Molecular mechanisms of acrolein toxicity: Relevance to human disease. Toxicological Sciences. 2015;**143**:242-255

[54] Kippler M, Tofail F, Gardner R, et al. Maternal cadmium exposure during pregnancy and size at birth: A prospective cohort study. Environmental Health Perspectives. 2012;**120**:284-289

[55] Rani A, Kumar A, Lal A, et al. Cellular mechanisms of cadmium-induced toxicity: A review. International Journal of Environmental Health Research. 2014;**24**:378-399

[56] Jin T, Lu J, Nordberg M. Toxicokinetics and biochemistry of cadmium with special emphasis on the role of metallothionein. Neurotoxicology. 1998;**19**:529-535

[57] De Mattia G, Bravi MC, Laurenti O, et al. Impairment of cell and plasma redox state in subjects professionally exposed to chromium. American Journal of Industrial Medicine. 2004;**46**:120-125

[58] Fowles J, Bates M, Noiton D. The Chemical Constituents in Cigarettes and Cigarette Smoke: Priorities for Harm Reduction: A Report to the New Zealand Ministry of Health. In: Jefferson F, Michael B. Epidemiology and Toxicology Group ESR: Kenepuru Science Centre; 2000

[59] LoPachin RM, Gavin T. Molecular mechanisms of aldehyde toxicity: A chemical perspective. Chemical Research in Toxicology. 2014;**27**:1081-1091

[60] Centers for Disease Control and Prevention. Nicotine: Systemic Agent. Available from: www.cdc.gov/niosh/ershdb/emergencyresponsecard_29750028.html [Accessed: 12 June 2017. Date last updated: 9 November 2017]

[61] England LJ, Bunnell RE, Pechacek TF, et al. Nicotine and the developing human: A neglected element in the electronic cigarette debate. American Journal of Preventive Medicine. 2015;**49**:286-293

[62] Kovacic P, Cooksy A. Iminium metabolite mechanism for nicotine toxicity and addiction: Oxidative stress and electron transfer. Medical Hypotheses. 2005;**64**:104-111

[63] Hebels DG, Briedé JJ, Khampang R, et al. Radical mechanisms in nitrosamine- and nitrosamide-induced whole-genome gene expression modulations in Caco-2 cells. Toxicological Sciences. 2010;**116**:194-205

[64] Rosenberg NL, Spitz MC, Filley CM, et al. Central nervous system effects of chronic toluene abuse—Clinical, brainstem evoked response and magnetic resonance imaging studies. Neurotoxicology and Teratology. 1988;**10**:489-495

[65] Cruz SL, Rivera-García MT, Woodward JJ. Review of toluene action: Clinical evidence, animal studies and molecular targets. Journal Drug Alcohol Research. 2014;**3**:235840

[66] Wani AL, Ara A, Usmani JA. Lead toxicity: A review. Interdisciplinary Toxicology. 2015;**8**:55-64

[67] Flora G, Gupta D, Tiwari A. Toxicity of lead: A review with recent updates. Interdisciplinary Toxicology. 2012;**5**:47-58

[68] Modi S, Sangani R, Alhajhusain A. Acute lipoid pneumonia secondary to e-cigarettes use: An unlikely replacement for cigarettes. Chest. 2015;**148**:382A

[69] Thornton S, Oller L, Sawyer T. Fatal intravenous injection of electronic eLiquid solution. Journal of Medical Toxicology. 2014;**10**:202-204

[70] Roger JM, Abayon M, Elad S, Kolokythas A. Oral trauma and tooth avulsion following explosion of e-cigarette. Journal of Oral and Maxillofacial Surgery. 2016;**74**:1181-1185

[71] Franck C, Filion KB, Kimmelman J, Grad R, Eisenberg MJ. Ethical considerations of e-cigarette use for tobacco harm reduction. Respiratory Research. 2016;**17**:53

[72] Saitta D, Ferro GA, Polosa R. Achieving appropriate regulations for electronic cigarettes. Therapeutic Advances in Chronic Disease. 2014;**5**:50-61

Chapter 3

Pain Associated with the Use of Electronic Cigarettes

Linda Tang

Abstract

Hitherto, lots of efforts have been made to illustrate the consequence of consuming conventional cigarette. The relationship between its utilization and the occurrence, deterioration, and variation of pain has been demonstrated for decades. As a result, electronic cigarette was investigated for its harmless and ideal replacement for conventional cigarette. Proposed and endorsed for almost 15 years, e-cigarette has established its success and induced many consumers. Later on, with greater attention to the increasing population indulging in or switching to electronic cigarette, complaints and side effects occurred and accumulated. Betwixt, headache, chest pain, thermal injury, withdrawal symptoms, and chronic pain had been described either via case reports or by experimental or clinical researches. Through comprehensively reviewing current publications, this chapter illustrates respective pain. With the introduction of this chapter, it will be helpful for the general public to understand the potential health implications of using e-cigarettes and evoke the readers' interest to learn more about this topic.

Keywords: electronic cigarette, conventional cigarette, pain, nicotine, thermal injury, withdrawal symptoms

1. Introduction

The harmful health and environmental implications of conventional cigarettes have been firmly established after decades of studies. Researchers and scientists have been engaged in unearthing and asserting their adverse effects. With the corporation of academic associations and governments, guidelines and law enforcements for cigarette control and management have achieved great success. However, because of the addiction to cigarette (mainly caused by nicotine, a pivotal component of conventional cigarette), it is challenging to propose a smooth transition period for smokers who want to quit. The emergence of electronic cigarettes (EC) greatly solved this issue for a short time and it became a dramatically successful approach for a period of time. More and more researchers assumed EC's harmlessness compared to conventional cigarette, since it is designed as an ideal replacement of conventional cigarette. But in the meanwhile, potential harmful consequences were found among adolescent and pregnant women who attempted to utilize or had been exposed to e-cigarette [1, 2]. The prevalent utilization of electronic cigarette has become a controversial topic and people hold contrasting opinions. On the one hand, American Cancer Society and Benowitz et al. hold its positive attitude toward EC because of its comparative less side-effect and well-behaved tolerance [3, 4]. On the other hand, accumulated evidence further expose the increasingly serious side effect of EC products [5, 6]. As a war of words, EC may be better to consumers' health than conventional cigarette, but it still plays a bad role in deteriorating the cardiovascular system and causing chest pain, especially for those who are undergoing existing cardiovascular disease. Scientists need a fresh mind to think about how EC correlates with pain feeling for its consumers [7].

Electronic cigarettes (ECs) or e-cigarettes are battery-operated products designed to deliver nicotine (can be without) combined with other chemicals such as flavors. An internal heat source turns nicotine and other chemicals into vapor when inhaled by the user. The main components of an EC include a cartridge, a heating atomizer, and a battery. With current evidence, the ingredients in the cartridge, the heating process, and spontaneous explosion of battery have the potential to do harm and cause pain to human beings [8–10]. Compared with pain caused by conventional cigarette, thermally induced pain is an emerging concern and effective preventative methods have not been developed yet [9–11]. Owing to its unpredictability, caution should be taken when carrying or vaping EC.

Finally, EC has grasped considerable public attention since 2014 based on the publication data of PubMed released. With relatively few years of investigation, neither the benefits nor the adverse effects of electronic cigarettes could be fully unearthed. Currently, the association between EC and various pains mainly depends on case reports and clinical questionnaire studies [12–14]. In this chapter, a systematic review will be conducted regarding both the common pains that EC consumers complained about using abundant data and the rare discomforts based on occasional cases. Moreover, a comprehensive comparison between conventional cigarette users and EC users can effectively demonstrate the potential effects of EC consumption, no matter first, second, or third hand.

2. Methods

Publications searching was conducted using PubMed and EMBASE with keywords: "electronic cigarette" or "e-cigarette" or "electronic nicotine delivery systems" or "vaping" or "tobacco products" or "cigarette smoking" and "pain" or "ache" or "musculoskeletal pain" or "chronic pain" or "headache" or "injury" without requirement of released time for the articles. All articles were written in English. All abstracts had been reviewed; if they met the topic of relationship between EC and pain, full-length articles were checked.

3. Headache

Headache is a symptom that could happen in any part of the brain with different mechanisms and in various ways. Based on an international online questionnaire study with large numbers of participants aiming to investigate the side effects and potential benefits of EC, headache was reported by 11.4% of who currently or previously consumed EC products [5]. It is worth mentioning that, for those participants who used EC, the concentration of nicotine was varied. Electronic cigarettes provide a gradual nicotine reduction strategy for those smokers who want to quit conventional smoking. According to this survey, there was no clear relationship between the frequency and severity of adverse effects and nicotine absorbed [5]. In an open-labeled, randomized, parallel group, clinical trial study was conducted at a certain nicotine concentration to probe the comparison between conventional smokers who switched to EC and those who continued with conventional cigarette for over 12 weeks. Researchers found no significant health improvement among those who switched, but rather adverse effects such as headaches and some other agonies, especially during the first week, and these symptoms could partially be ascribed to nicotine withdrawal [15]. Later on, the same participants participated in a trial that wanted to evaluate the long-term effects of EC consumption; after 24 months of investigation, the study showed that headache was the most complained symptom and there were no worse clinical presentation compared with the baseline condition [12]. Similarly, systems that retrospectively reviewed and summarized the recent clinical complications of using EC found that headache was actually the most frequently reported adverse effect [16].

Headache, either associated with nicotine withdrawal symptoms or unknown mechanisms, could impressively prevent smokers to quit conventional smoking and switch to low-harmful EC products. In the studies shown above, there were no details on how the headaches happened nor its frequency and severity. Furthermore, some of the clinical studies were mainly based on online questionnaires; thus, there could have been selection bias and the criteria might have been interpreted more subjectively than objectively. More studies are needed in both experimental and clinical fields.

4. Chest pain

Among those e-cigarette-using individuals who complained about chest pain, the most reported syndromes were related with either lung malfunction, structure disfigures [17, 18], or potential cardiovascular diseases [19].

Consistent evidence has shown that conventional cigarette users are readily trapped in lung problems. However, only a limited number of studies have focused on EC users who caught chest pain. Dr. Sommerfeld et al.'s study [17] presented a previously healthy young woman who developed pleuritic chest pain after EC use. Soon the chest pain deteriorated into acute respiratory distress syndrome after acute respiratory failure. With completed routine and pathological examination, this patient was diagnosed with hypersensitivity pneumonitis after using EC products with unknown mechanism. This particular case reminds clinicians and consumers of EC's rare but dreadful consequences. Another patient was a previous conventional cigarette consumer who switched to EC to quit smoking. A month later, this patient was referred to the pulmonary department and complained about a month-long pain that was sharp, intermittent, and on both sides of the chest. Upon inpatient studies, dyspnea was confirmed and the doctors ascribed her symptoms to the recent EC use. Later, she was diagnosed with organizing pneumonia via pathological examination and was improved with steroids along with abstinence from e-cigarette use [18]. This case demonstrated that EC contributes to the deterioration of patients' health and possibly causes chest pain through various mechanisms. According to an international survey, about 3% of EC users have struggled with chest pain [5]. Even without thoroughly investigating the disadvantages of EC, attention should be paid when EC is used without other choices.

Nicotine, the major component of conventional cigarette, was ascertained to induce addiction, which impedes smokers to quit conventional cigarette by causing difficult withdrawal symptoms [1, 8]. This leads to the rise of electronic cigarettes, designed to help quit smoking with less withdrawal agony. Its designer claimed that it is the ideal replacement for conventional cigarette but with much less nicotine inside. But when surveys were conducted to clarify the components of EC, the concentration of nicotine varied among different brands and products [4]. A randomized, partially single-blinded, 6-period crossover clinical study of adult smokers was conducted to compare how nicotine alteration impacts smoking urge between EC users and conventional cigarette users. Though obvious blood plasma nicotine levels were detected, subjects who were exposed to EC products behaved better than conventional cigarette users [20]. On the other hand, holding alternative opinion toward the advantage of using EC, Lee et al. [21] demonstrated that smoking electronic cigarettes could damage DNA and reduce repair activity in mouse lung, heart, and bladder via various chemical measurements and predicted its harm in human lung and bladder cells [21].

With regard to cardiovascular symptoms induced by EC, the mainstream opinion is mostly positive because it is relatively harmless compared with conventional cigarette [3, 4, 7]. However, consumers should be cautious that smoking EC is not totally free of danger as cases have shown EC users develop cardiovascular diseases, especially among young people and women who are pregnant [4, 7]. Based on experimental studies, EC components have the potential to activate platelet activation, adhesion, inflammation, and aggregation, which are critical steps for the occurrence and development of cardiovascular diseases [22]. The unfavorable influence of EC has also been demonstrated on young smokers who were previously free of cardiovascular diseases. The researchers suggested that using EC can increase aortic stiffness and blood pressure in addition to the unfavorable effect on the cardiovascular system [19].

Chest pain seems to be caused less frequently and less seriously with EC consumption than with conventional cigarette usage. However, due to shortage of investigation, no conclusive statement about its harm could be drawn. To summarize, EC users still encounter various kinds of chest pain; among them, chest pain induced by cardiovascular system is relatively specific and likely caused by the effects of nicotine [7, 20], while, for other chest pains that are mainly ascribed to respiratory system malfunction, acute pain was prone to happen and is probably correlated with hyper-immune response [5, 17, 18].

5. Other specific pains

There are still other specific pains reported as a consequence of EC consumption. Such aches mainly occurred in the abdomen [23] and the oral cavity [24].

Dr. Madsen et al. reported a 45-year-old female who presented with abdominal pain and fever, conceivably caused by inflammatory reaction after abrupt EC use. Imaging evidence suggested lung cancer metastasis, while pathological examination was negative for malignant findings and suggested a foreign body reaction. Upon cessation of e-cigarette use, this patient made a recovery. This was a unique case leading inflammatory reaction of EC to mimic metastatic cancer [23].

A cross-sectional study aimed to investigate the relationship between EC use and oral health among adolescents showed that EC use possibly increased the risk of tongue and inside-cheek pain among student users in Korea [24]. Specific to this study, gingival pain was not found significantly more frequent when compared with the non-EC group [24]. However, an international questionnaire survey suggested that 13.1% of EC users developed gingivitis in about a 10-month follow-up [5]. Some have tried to explain the difference in findings by considering ethnic differences or ways of vaping.

Reported occasionally and lacking profound investigation, these aches were possibly correlated with EC use. Likewise, EC caused chest pain through induced inflammatory reaction [17] and induced abdominal pain via a similar mechanism [23]. For oral pain, inconsistent results were obtained from surveys. Gingival pain did occur more frequently among EC users even though there were no complete statistical agreements. More studies and surveys should be conducted to address this issue.

6. Thermal injury

Thermal injury hardly happens during conventional cigarette use. However, due to the instability of device and improper carrying methods, both physical and chemical exposure could happen to EC users. There seems to be no effective way to prevent thermal injury other than quitting. Most recent thermal injury cases reported were associated with the explosion of battery or high-temperature vaping [9–11, 25, 26]. Since a considerable number of cases and researches concluded that EC use is responsible for thermal pain, greater public attention is needed.

Paley et al. [25] reported two cases in which the explosion of EC products caused corneoscleral laceration and ocular burns and such effects were like nightmares for the patients and their family. Through retrospectively reviewing the institutional burn database of EC injury, Serror et al. [9] illustrated the potential mechanism underlying thermal EC injury. They reached four possible mechanisms: (1) thermal burns by flames due to a phenomenon called "thermal runaway," (2) blast lesions secondary to the explosion, (3) chemical alkali burns caused by the spread of the electrolyte solution, and (4) thermal burns without flames due to overheating. Their results provide a way to redesign and improve the safety of EC devices. Meanwhile, another retrospective survey was conducted to investigate the severity of pain those patients suffered; they concluded that the majority of EC explosions caused second- and third-degree burns within the same wound bed. Among those who got injured, the spontaneous explosion of the battery was the most common reason. Explosion of these products also occasionally made an unbearable impact on spine and caused C1 and C2 fractures in a young EC user. Data collected from the US Consumer Product Safety Commission's National Electronic Injury Surveillance System revealed more explosion and burn injuries recently [11].

Thermal injury is increasingly threatening to those EC users who are not cautious; incidents that occurred can actually cause a serious condition and victims should be referred to emergency treatment. The critical point is thermal injury seems unpredictable without suitable regulation of these devices since it can happen spontaneously.

7. Withdrawal symptoms and chronic pain

Withdrawal symptoms should mainly be attributed to nicotine, a miraculous compound that causes addictive feeling and prevents current smokers from quitting. Withdrawal symptoms are a series of discomforts arisen owing to the short of nicotine. To investigate the pain behavior in smokers and non-smokers, experiments unearthed that smoking withdrawal was associated with blunted stress response and increased pain sensitivity [27]. This finding suggests that during the time when smokers are trying to quit cigarette consumption, they will suffer more pain sensitivity and consequently be unable to keep up with the process. The same story is revealed by an online survey that aimed to test the association between pain and the potential to quit smoking. They found that smokers who suffered chronic pain had less willingness, lower confidence, and greater difficulty to quit cigarette [28]. Moreover, based on a rat model, nicotine deprivation (which produces a similar mechanism as nicotine withdrawal) increased the pain threshold and decreased the pain tolerance [29]. Along the same lines, researches revealed that pain severity was significantly and positively associated with e-cigarette dependence [6, 13]. These experiments had demonstrated the relationship between pain-taking and the possibility of getting rid of nicotine-based cigarette.

Consistent and severe pain feeling caused by withdrawal syndrome was the most critical problem that hampered users to quit tobacco products. Even though EC products claimed to have less nicotine, they still arouse ache among EC consumers, especially for those who used conventional and electronic cigarette at the same time. Most pains were unspecific for those individuals who complained about withdrawal symptoms, which had no simple approaches to cure. As a consequence, chronic pains in withdrawal symptoms correlate with EC usage; it cannot be neglected and should be taken into serious consideration.

8. Compounds and potential pains

Aerosol and e-liquid are the major components of EC products that are mixed with various ingredients [3]. The process of vaping can produce some heavy metal contamination to smokers and second-hand or third-hand delivered harm. Though few researches have been done to interpret the side effects of EC, experimental studies illustrate the effects of some chemicals. Through reflection X-ray fluorescence spectroscopy, aldehydes, cadmium, lead, nickel, copper, arsenic, and chromium were detected in different types of EC products and they are likely to be harmful to human health [30].

Studies using ALDH2*1/*2 heterozygous mice, designed to be impaired in the metabolic aldehydes, found they were significantly more sensitive to painful stimuli than other wild-type mice and this alteration can be inhibited by an ALDH2-selective activator [31]. This experiment proposed the possibility of aldehydes altering the threshold of pain. Furthermore, EC users are possibly exposed to toluene and formalin owing to vaping. Cervantes-Duran et al. [32] suggested that acute toluene exposure fomented formalin-induced acute and long-lasting nociceptive hypersensitivity in rats [32]. Meanwhile, propylene glycol could attenuate the adverse effects of high-dose nicotine and allow EC users to develop high tolerance toward EC products [33]. By analyzing urinary cadmium levels, La-Up et al. [34] found there was a positive relationship between urinary cadmium level and chronic musculoskeletal pain. The survey showed that for the cadmium-contaminated areas in northwest Thailand, people had high risk of being trapped in chronic musculoskeletal pain. This finding in turn suggests that exposure to cadmium, which is contained in EC vaping, may cause chronic musculoskeletal pain [34].

All in all, the compounds in EC products vary. Some of them are found in conventional cigarettes while others are newly discovered. A large amount of these compounds have the potential to alter pain threshold or induce pain feeling. Until recently, the cause mechanism was not fully illustrated and individuals are still exposed to false advertisements and potential second- or third-hand vaping. Such conditions are partially caused by the lack of clear quality control and quality assurance, since different EC products could have different ingredients.

9. Conclusion

Electronic cigarettes, once considered an ideal replacement of conventional cigarette for current smokers, have caused considerable problems and grasped public and researchers' attention recently. First of all, EC products are not harmless [3, 5] and EC consumers have not fully understood the potential harms of EC usage yet

[1, 4]. In addition, even with a limited number of studies, lots of researches were conducted to compare conventional cigarette and EC; their findings agreed that EC does have its disadvantages and the relationship between EC use and pain is still on its way to become fully clarified.

The apparent safety of EC appeals to current conventional cigarette users, who consider using it to help them avoid the dreadful consequences of cigarette consumption [6]. Meanwhile, EC also allows youngsters to satisfy their curiosity without violating the law and without causing obvious health concerns compared to conventional cigarette (at least before major health and environmental concerns are brought to public attention). Thanks to the enthusiasm on investigating EC and recent findings, stricter prohibition of EC usage in public areas and better prevention of EC exposure to youngsters and women have been enacted [14].

Above all, consuming EC products does have its harm toward human health, though it is relatively safe compared with conventional cigarette usage [3, 4]. EC consumption has possibly led to headache [5, 12, 15], chest pain [5, 17], thermal injury [10, 11], and other pain-related agonies. Fortunately, scientists have begun to test EC components more thoroughly and are trying to conclude the adverse effects of EC consumption.

While the discussion of EC's advantage and disadvantage is still fierce and there is still uncertainty about mechanism and the prevalence of pain, researches and clinical cases will reach a comprehensive evaluation of EC with growing evidence.

Author details

Linda Tang
Duke University, Durham, United States

*Address all correspondence to: lyt3@duke.edu

References

[1] Protano C, Di Milia LM, Orsi GB, Vitali M. Electronic cigarette: A threat or an opportunity for public health? State of the art and future perspectives. La Clinica Terapeutica. 2015;**166**(1): 32-37

[2] Wang TW, Marynak KL, Agaku IT, King BA. Secondhand exposure to electronic cigarette aerosol among us youths. JAMA Pediatrics. 2017;**171**(5): 490-492

[3] Drope J, Cahn Z, Kennedy R, Liber AC, Stoklosa M, Henson R, et al. Key issues surrounding the health impacts of electronic nicotine delivery systems (ENDS) and other sources of nicotine. CA: A Cancer Journal for Clinicians. 2017;**67**(6):449-471

[4] Benowitz NL, Fraiman JB. Cardiovascular effects of electronic cigarettes. Nature Reviews Cardiology. 2017;**14**(8):447-456

[5] Farsalinos KE, Romagna G, Tsiapras D, Kyrzopoulos S, Voudris V. Characteristics, perceived side effects and benefits of electronic cigarette use: A worldwide survey of more than 19,000 consumers. International Journal of Environmental Research and Public Health. 2014;**11**(4):4356-4373

[6] Zvolensky MJ, Garey L, Mayorga NA, Rogers AH, Orr MF, Ditre JW, et al. Current pain severity and electronic cigarettes: An initial empirical investigation. Journal of Behavioral Medicine. 2018

[7] Qasim H, Karim ZA, Rivera JO, Khasawneh FT, Alshbool FZ. Impact of electronic cigarettes on the cardiovascular system. Journal of the American Heart Association. 2017;**6**(9): e006353

[8] Rom O, Pecorelli A, Valacchi G, Reznick AZ. Are e-cigarettes a safe and good alternative to cigarette smoking? Annals of the New York Academy of Sciences. 2015;**1340**:65-74

[9] Serror K, Chaouat M, Legrand MM, Depret F, Haddad J, Malca N, et al. Burns caused by electronic vaping devices (e-cigarettes): A new classification proposal based on mechanisms. Burns: Journal of the International Society for Burn Injuries. 2018;**44**(3):544-548

[10] Hickey S, Goverman J, Friedstat J, Sheridan R, Schulz J. Thermal injuries from exploding electronic cigarettes. Burns: Journal of the International Society for Burn Injuries. 2018;**44**(5): 1294-1301

[11] Rossheim ME, Livingston MD, Soule EK, Zeraye HA, Thombs DL. Electronic cigarette explosion and burn injuries, US emergency departments 2015–2017. Tobacco Control. 2018

[12] Walele T, Bush J, Koch A, Savioz R, Martin C, O'Connell G. Evaluation of the safety profile of an electronic vapour product used for two years by smokers in a real-life setting. Regulatory Toxicology and Pharmacology: RTP. 2018;**92**:226-238

[13] Kosiba JD, Zale EL, Ditre JW. Associations between pain intensity and urge to smoke: Testing the role of negative affect and pain catastrophizing. Drug and Alcohol Dependence. 2018;**187**:100-108

[14] Mitchell MD, Mannino DM, Steinke DT, Kryscio RJ, Bush HM, Crofford LJ. Association of smoking and chronic pain syndromes in Kentucky women. The Journal of Pain: Official Journal of the American Pain Society. 2011;**12**(8): 892-899

[15] Cravo AS, Bush J, Sharma G, Savioz R, Martin C, Craige S, et al. A

randomised, parallel group study to evaluate the safety profile of an electronic vapour product over 12 weeks. Regulatory Toxicology and Pharmacology: RTP. 2016;**81**(Supp. 1): S1-S14

[16] Gualano MR, Passi S, Bert F, La Torre G, Scaioli G, Siliquini R. Electronic cigarettes: Assessing the efficacy and the adverse effects through a systematic review of published studies. Journal of Public Health (Oxford, England). 2015;**37**(3):488-497

[17] Sommerfeld CG, Weiner DJ, Nowalk A, Larkin A. Hypersensitivity pneumonitis and acute respiratory distress syndrome from E-cigarette use. Pediatrics. 2018;**141**(6):e20163927

[18] Khan MS, Khateeb F, Akhtar J, Khan Z, Lal A, Kholodovych V, et al. Organizing pneumonia related to electronic cigarette use: A case report and review of literature. The Clinical Respiratory Journal. 2018;**12**(3): 1295-1299

[19] Vlachopoulos C, Ioakeimidis N, Abdelrasoul M, Terentes-Printzios D, Georgakopoulos C, Pietri P, et al. Electronic cigarette smoking increases aortic stiffness and blood pressure in young smokers. Journal of the American College of Cardiology. 2016;**67**(23): 2802-2803

[20] D'Ruiz CD, Graff DW, Yan XS. Nicotine delivery, tolerability and reduction of smoking urge in smokers following short-term use of one brand of electronic cigarettes. BMC Public Health. 2015;**15**:991

[21] Lee HW, Park SH, Weng MW, Wang HT, Huang WC, Lepor H, et al. E-cigarette smoke damages DNA and reduces repair activity in mouse lung, heart, and bladder as well as in human lung and bladder cells. Proceedings of the National Academy of Sciences of the United States of America. 2018;**115**(7): E1560-E1569

[22] Hom S, Chen L, Wang T, Ghebrehiwet B, Yin W, Rubenstein DA. Platelet activation, adhesion, inflammation, and aggregation potential are altered in the presence of electronic cigarette extracts of variable nicotine concentrations. Platelets. 2016;**27**(7): 694-702

[23] Ring Madsen L, Vinther Krarup NH, Bergmann TK, Baerentzen S, Neghabat S, Duval L, et al. A cancer that went up in smoke: Pulmonary reaction to e-cigarettes imitating metastatic cancer. Chest. 2016;**149**(3):e65-e67

[24] Cho JH. The association between electronic-cigarette use and self-reported oral symptoms including cracked or broken teeth and tongue and/or inside-cheek pain among adolescents: A cross-sectional study. PLoS One. 2017; **12**(7):e0180506

[25] Paley GL, Echalier E, Eck TW, Hong AR, Farooq AV, Gregory DG, et al. Corneoscleral laceration and ocular burns caused by electronic cigarette explosions. Cornea. 2016;**35**(7): 1015-1018

[26] Norii T, Plate A. Electronic cigarette explosion resulting in a C1 and C2 fracture: A case report. The Journal of Emergency Medicine. 2017;**52**(1):86-88

[27] Nakajima M, Al'Absi M. Nicotine withdrawal and stress-induced changes in pain sensitivity: A cross-sectional investigation between abstinent smokers and nonsmokers. Psychophysiology. 2014;**51**(10): 1015-1022

[28] Ditre JW, Kosiba JD, Zale EL, Zvolensky MJ, Maisto SA. Chronic pain status, nicotine withdrawal, and expectancies for smoking cessation among lighter smokers. Annals of Behavioral Medicine. 2016;**50**(3): 427-435

[29] Baiamonte BA, Stickley SC, Ford SJ. Nicotine deprivation produces deficits

in pain perception that are moderately attenuated by caffeine consumption. Journal of Psychoactive Drugs. 2016; **48**(3):159-165

[30] Kamilari E, Farsalinos K, Poulas K, Kontoyannis CG, Orkoula MG. Detection and quantitative determination of heavy metals in electronic cigarette refill liquids using total reflection X-ray fluorescence spectrometry. Food and Chemical Toxicology. 2018;**116**(Pt B):233-237

[31] Zambelli VO, Gross ER, Chen CH, Gutierrez VP, Cury Y, Mochly-Rosen D. Aldehyde dehydrogenase-2 regulates nociception in rodent models of acute inflammatory pain. Science Translational Medicine. 2014;**6**(251): 251ra118

[32] Cervantes-Duran C, Ortega-Varela LF, Godinez-Hernandez D, Granados-Soto V, Gauthereau-Torres MY. Toluene exposure enhances acute and chronic formalin-induced nociception in rats: Participation of 5-HT3 receptors. Neurotoxicology. 2017;**63**:97-105

[33] Harris AC, Muelken P, Haave Z, Swain Y, Smethells JR, LeSage MG. Propylene glycol, a major electronic cigarette constituent, attenuates the adverse effects of high-dose nicotine as measured by intracranial self-stimulation in rats. Drug and Alcohol Dependence. 2018;**193**:162-168

[34] La-Up A, Wiwatanadate P, Uthaikhup S, Pruenglampoo S. Association between urinary cadmium and chronic musculoskeletal pain in residents of cadmium-contaminated area in Northwest Thailand. Environmental Science and Pollution Research International. 2018;**25**(14): 14182-14187

Chapter 4

Regulation of Electronic Cigarettes in the United States

Azim Chowdhury

Abstract

In the United States, the manufacture, distribution and marketing of tobacco products is regulated by the US Food and Drug Administration (FDA), pursuant to authority extended to the agency in 2009 with the enactment of the Family Smoking Prevention and Tobacco Control Act (Tobacco Control Act). While that law initially gave FDA authority over certain categories of tobacco products (e.g., cigarettes, smokeless tobacco and roll-your-own tobacco), in August 2016, FDA's "Deeming Rule" extended that authority to all products that are made from or contain tobacco-derived substances, such as nicotine. Now, products such as cigars, pipe tobacco, shisha/hookah and electronic cigarettes (e-cigarettes) are subject to the Tobacco Control Act and FDA's authority. But regulators have struggled to keep up with the evolving technology and are still grappling with the public health consequences—both pro and con—and continue to adopt policies and regulations to address new issues that emerge (i.e., underage use and flavors).

Keywords: FDA, e-cigarette, tobacco, nicotine, Deeming, Tobacco Control Act, flavors, PMTA, premarket review, continuum of risk

1. Introduction

The emergence of less risky novel or "next generation" tobacco products such as e-cigarettes and heat-not-burn devices coincided with new regulatory authority provided to the US Food and Drug Administration (FDA), the health agency in charge of regulating the safety of consumer products such as food, drugs, medical devices, and cosmetics, under the Family Smoking Prevention and Tobacco Control Act (Tobacco Control Act), which amended the existing Food, Drug, and Cosmetic Act (FDCA or Act). Pursuant to this new law, FDA now has the authority to regulate the manufacture, distribution, and marketing of tobacco products in the United States [1].

When it was signed into law in June 2009, the Tobacco Control Act provided FDA with immediate authority only over four categories of tobacco products, that is, cigarettes, cigarette tobacco, smokeless tobacco, and roll-your-own tobacco. Subsequently, in 2016, FDA finalized its "Deeming Rule," 81 Fed. Reg. 28974 (May 10, 2016), which deemed *all* products that meet the tobacco product definition (including, but not limited to, e-cigarettes, heat-not-burn, cigars, hookah/waterpipe, and pipe tobacco products) to be subject to its Tobacco Control Act authority. Now, newly deemed products are subject to a host of federal requirements including, among other things, premarket authorization for new products, ingredient reporting, manufacturing establishment registration, harmful constituent testing, and sales and marketing restrictions.

Rising underage use of e-cigarettes has underscored the need for increased FDA enforcement of the Tobacco Control Act requirements, and has resulted in new policies aimed at restricted youth access to flavored e-cigarettes. This paper provides a comprehensive review of the regulatory requirements applicable to manufacturers and addresses how FDA's most recent policy announcements could impact the industry moving forward.

2. Overview of major Tobacco Control Act requirements

The Tobacco Control Act requires tobacco product manufacturers to, among other things, register their US manufacturing establishments with FDA, submit a list of US manufactured products, report the ingredients used in their products, submit certain health documents in their possession, test their products for specific harmful and potentially harmful constituents (HPHCs), include nicotine addiction warnings and certain other information on their labels and, most critically, obtain premarket authorization for any new products. Manufacturers are also subject to the adulteration and misbranding provision of the Act and are prohibited from making modified risk claims about their products without specific FDA authorization.

2.1 Marketing and sales restrictions

With respect to the sales and marketing of deemed products, FDA's Deeming Rule bans claims of reduced or "modified" risk and free samples to consumers, sets the minimum purchase age to 18 years, requires photo-ID verification at the point-of-sale, restricts vending machine sales of covered tobacco products to adult-only facilities, and requires nicotine addiction warnings on labels and advertising [2]. Furthermore, it is illegal to market or distribute any tobacco product whose packaging or labeling is misbranded under Section 903 of the FDCA, or deceptive and misleading under Section 5 of the Federal Trade Commission (FTC) Act.

2.2 US establishment registration and product listing

Section 905(b) of the Tobacco Control Act requires every person who owns or operates any establishment in the United States that manufactures, prepares, compounds, or processes finished tobacco products to register such establishment with FDA and submit a product list, which must be updated biannually (every December 31 and June 30) [3]. Foreign establishments are not presently required to register with FDA, but the agency has the authority to promulgate a regulation requiring them to do so. Here, the phrase "manufacture, preparation, compounding, or processing" includes repackaging or otherwise changing the container, wrapper, or labeling of any tobacco product package in furtherance of the distribution of the tobacco product. US importers of tobacco products do not register with FDA unless they are also engaged in a manufacturing activity in the United States.

As noted, at the time of registration, registrants must submit to FDA a detailed list of all products that are being manufactured, prepared, compounded, or processed for commercial distribution in the United States, along with all labeling, and a representative sampling of advertisements. The term "commercial distribution" includes any distribution of a tobacco product to consumers or to another person for further manufacturing through sale or otherwise [4]. Registrants must also file a biannual report of certain changes to their product lists [5].

Registered establishments are subject to FDA inspection every 2 years [6]. FDA may inspect factories, warehouses, and other establishments in which tobacco products are manufactured, processed, packed, or held, as well as any vehicle being used to transport or hold such products [7].

2.3 Ingredient reporting

Section 904(a)(1)-(2) of the Tobacco Control Act requires that a manufacturer or importer submit a listing of all ingredients, as well as a description of the content, delivery, and form of nicotine in each tobacco product [8]. "Ingredients" here includes "tobacco, substances, compounds, and additives" [9]—that are added to any component or part of the products (e.g., to the tobacco, paper, filter, or other part). Products must be identified by brand and sub-brand and the ingredients by quantity in each brand and sub-brand. Manufacturers and importers are also required to submit information whenever any additive, or the quantity of any additive, is changed [10]. This requirement applies to all manufacturers no matter where they are located.

However, on April 13, 2018, FDA published a Revised Guidance for Industry which clarified that, at this time, FDA is effectively exempting e-cigarette device and hardware component/part manufacturers from the ingredient listing requirement [11]. Rather, FDA only intends to enforce the Section 904 ingredient listing requirement with respect to those tobacco products that are (1) made or derived from tobacco, or (2) made with *consumable* ingredients that are burned, aerosolized or ingested when the tobacco product is being used. Specifically, for e-cigarettes, FDA is now only seeking ingredient information on e-liquids, and **not** any hardware or components/parts such as:

- Electrical components including, but not limited to, batteries, charging systems, circuit boards, wiring, and connectors
- System software
- Digital display, lights, and buttons to adjust settings
- Connection adapters
- Cartomizers
- Coils
- Wicks
- Tanks
- Mouthpieces

2.4 Reporting health documents

Section 904 obligates tobacco product manufacturers and importers to submit certain health information to FDA. Specifically, manufacturers and importers are also required to submit all documents relating to the health, toxicological, behavioral, or physiologic effects of current or future tobacco products, constituents, ingredients, components, and additives (collectively, "Health Documents"). The term "documents" is defined broadly and includes "writings, drawings, graphs, charts, photographs, sound recordings, images, and other data or data compilations—stored in any medium from which information can be obtained either directly or, if necessary, after translation by the responding party into a reasonably usable form." At this time, however, FDA is only requesting health documents developed between June 23, 2009 and December 31, 2009. Companies that may not have been in business, or who were not producing health documents on their tobacco products at that time, are still required to notify FDA that they do not have any relevant health documents in their possession [12].

2.5 Harmful constituent testing

Section 904(a)(3) requires manufacturers and importers to report quantities of HPHCs found in tobacco products or tobacco smoke by brand and sub-brand. Out of more than 7000 such constituents, FDA has established a list of 93 HPHCs that tobacco companies will ultimately be required to report for every regulated tobacco product sold in the USA [13]. However, in recognition of current testing limitations for certain constituents on FDA's list, FDA has created representative or "abbreviated" lists of constituents for cigarettes, roll-your-own, and smokeless tobacco for which testing methods are well established and widely available [14].

With respect to e-cigarettes, as of the date of this writing, FDA has not provided any guidance or initiated rulemaking, so it is unclear whether HPHCs will need to be tested in the e-liquids themselves or in the vapor/aerosol formed when used in a device. In August 2016 FDA published a revised guidance document expanding the definition of HPHC to specifically include substances in the vapor (aerosol) produced by e-cigarettes. As defined by FDA in the guidance, an HPHC now includes any chemical or chemical compound in a tobacco product or in tobacco smoke that: (a) is, or potentially is, inhaled, ingested, or absorbed into the body, including as an aerosol (vapor) or any other emission; and (b) causes or has the potential to cause direct or indirect harm to users or non-users of tobacco products" [14].

FDA is expected to issue formal guidance and regulations for the testing and reporting of HPHCs, ingredients, additives and other constituents pursuant to Section 915 [15].

2.6 Label requirements

The Deeming Rule extended a number of labeling requirements to deemed tobacco products. Specifically, by August 10, 2018, all deemed tobacco products must include the following on the labels of all products marketed in the United States:

- The name and place of business of the manufacturer, packer, or distributor;
- An accurate statement of the quantity of the contents in terms of weight, measure, or numerical count; and
- The statement "Sale only allowed in the United States".

In addition, all nicotine-containing products must include the following warning on their labels "WARNING: This product contains nicotine. Nicotine is an addictive chemical" [16]. That warning label must comply with the specific requirements set forth in 21 C.F.R. § 1143.3(a). The nicotine addiction warning requirement, however, does not apply to products that are not sold with or contain nicotine [17]. Rather, covered tobacco products that do not contain nicotine (i.e., zero-nicotine e-cigarettes that contain *another* tobacco-derived ingredient), must include the following statement on their label in lieu of the nicotine addiction warning: "This product is made from tobacco." Manufacturers of such products are further required to submit a statement to FDA certifying that the product does not contain nicotine.

2.7 Premarket authorization for new tobacco products

The Tobacco Control Act requires that FDA authorize the marketing of any new tobacco product through a lengthy and complicated application process. If a product was on the market as of February 15, 2007 it is considered "grandfathered" and exempt from FDA premarket review. If a tobacco product was introduced (or is intended to be introduced) after the February 15, 2007 "grandfather date," or if it was modified in any way after that date, it is a new product. Product modifications include, but are not limited to changes to a product's design, ingredients, components, parts, delivery mechanism, type of nicotine, etc. Changes to a product's labeling (including brand name, logos, colors, etc.), however, do not trigger the premarket review requirements [18].

The substantial equivalence (SE) report and the premarket tobacco application (PMTA) are the primary pathways for new tobacco product. The minor modification or SE exemption pathway is another option but only applies to changes in additives so is rarely utilized.

If a manufacturer can demonstrate, through the submission of an SE report, that its new product is substantially equivalent to a "predicate" product it may be authorized for sale. A "predicate" product is either a grandfathered tobacco product (that was on the market as of February 15, 2007), or tobacco product that, although not itself grandfathered, has been determined to be substantially equivalent to another grandfathered product. To demonstrate substantial equivalence, the manufacturer must provide evidence (such as data showing similarities in consumer perception, clinical data, abuse liability data, and toxicology) that the new product has the same (identical) "characteristics" as the predicate tobacco product or, if it has different characteristics, that the new product "does not raise different questions of public health." In other words, FDA may find a new tobacco product to be substantially equivalent to the identified predicate if the new characteristics do not create different public health concerns compared to the predicate. Public health concerns may include the potential to increase tobacco use initiation or decrease cessation.

For a PMTA, on the other hand, a predicate product is not needed. Rather, the manufacturer must demonstrate that the new product meets a very high public health standard. Specifically, it must be shown that the product, if made available in the United States, would be "appropriate for the protection of the public health." This requires assessing the product's potential impact on the population, including its impact on overall tobacco product cessation rates (i.e., the likelihood that people will stop using tobacco products), as well as initiation rates (i.e., the likelihood that people will start using tobacco products) [19].

To meet this high standard, FDA has recommended PMTAs include detailed scientific literature reviews, as well as numerous non-clinical, clinical (i.e., human), and long-term studies be performed, including, but not limited to, in-vitro and in-vivo (i.e., animal) toxicological studies (e.g., genotoxicity and cytotoxicity), as well as clinical and population-level studies to assess consumer perceptions, likelihood of initiation and cessation, product use patterns, abuse liability, and health outcomes [19].

2.7.1 Compliance policy for deemed tobacco products

As noted, in the final Deeming Rule FDA chose not to amend the February 15, 2007 grandfather date for deemed products, forcing *all* next generation products to go through pre-market authorization (because there are no known grandfathered e-cigarettes or heat-not-burn products). Moreover, as a result, the SE Report pathway (which, as noted above, requires a manufacturer to compare a new product to a predicate product) is unavailable, forcing all next generation products to go through the much more onerous and expensive PMTA.

FDA instead established a compliance policy that would allow any finished deemed tobacco product marketed after the grandfather date and prior to August 8, 2016 (the rule's effective date), to remain on the market for 2 years (without premarket authorization) until August 8, 2018, at which time PMTAs would need to be submitted. Products subject to such PMTAs that are accepted by FDA for review would be permitted to remain on the market for an additional year, until August 8, 2019 (the "sunset period"), at which point they would have to be removed from market and wait for FDA authorization (which, of course, is not guaranteed and could take years).

Lawsuits were filed challenging FDA's failure to change the grandfather date and the seemingly arbitrary 2-year PMTA compliance policy, and there has been an intense lobbying effort to get Congress to change the grandfather date—so far, to no avail [20].

However, on July 28, 2017, FDA announced a new "comprehensive regulatory plan to shift the trajectory of tobacco-related disease, death" that refocuses the agency's implementation of the Tobacco Control Act and the Deeming Rule [21]. While the focus of the announcement was to highlight the agency's long-term plan to potentially reduce nicotine in cigarettes to "non-addictive" levels, the agency also discussed the potential harm-reduction benefits of deemed products like e-cigarettes, and appeared to recognize that a "continuum of risk" of tobacco and nicotine-containing products exists.

In this regard, as part of its comprehensive policy announcement, FDA delayed the Deeming Rule's compliance policy deadlines to submit premarket authorization applications" (i.e., PMTAs or SE reports) for newly deemed tobacco products that were on the market on August 8, 2016. Under the new timelines, applications for previously marketed (but not grandfathered) combustible products, such as cigars, pipe tobacco and hookah tobacco, are now due by August 8, 2021, and applications for previously marketed non-combustibles, such as e-cigarettes, e-liquids and heat-not-burn products are due by August 8, 2022. FDA also indicated that it would be revising the sunset policy so that existing products under review can remain on the market pending review of their applications. New products intended to enter the market *after* August 8, 2016 must still obtain FDA marketing authorization *before* entering the market.

This new compliance policy delaying premarket review provided the industry, which was facing a de facto ban in 2018, much needed breathing room on the most complicated and expensive regulatory requirement. Critical to ensuring that such ban is not simply delayed until 2022 will depend, in part, on whether FDA provides more guidance and clarity on the PMTA process and requirements—particularly how to satisfy the population-level public health standard.

In addition to extending the premarket review deadlines for deemed products, FDA announced that it will publish advance notices of proposed rulemaking (ANPRMs) to seek (1) input on the potential public health benefits and possible adverse effects of lowering the level of nicotine in cigarettes to non-addictive levels, (2) public comments on the role of flavored tobacco products in terms of youth initiation and harm reduction, and (3) scientific data related to the patterns of use and resulting public health impacts from premium cigars. FDA also indicated that it would develop product standards to address public health risks, such as, e-cigarette battery safety issues, and exposure to liquid nicotine by children, as well as examine ways to increase access and use of FDA-approved medicinal nicotine products intended to help smokers quit [21].

2.8 New FDA policy to address increase in underage e-cigarette use

In April 2018 FDA launched its Youth Tobacco Prevention Plan to address the sudden rise in underage use of certain types of e-cigarettes: pre-filled cartridge-based e-cigarettes sold mainly in convenience stores, gas stations and similar all-age retail outlets. FDA stated that between June and September 2018 nearly 1300 retailers across the country had received warning letters and/or monetary penalties for selling products to minors [22]. FDA also requested manufacturers of these popular cartridge-based e-cigarettes to submit proposals on how they plan to curtail the increasing youth-use of their products.

Subsequently, on November 15, 2018, FDA announced a new policy aimed at preventing youth access to flavored e-cigarettes [23]. First, FDA announced that all flavored e-cigarette products (other than tobacco, mint, and menthol flavors, or non-flavored products) will be required to be sold in age-restricted, in-person locations, or else potentially be subjected to a revised premarket review compliance policy deadline. This policy revision would apply to all e-cigarettes, including e-liquids, cartridge-based systems and cigalikes, in flavors except tobacco, mint, and menthol, sold in physical locations where people under age 18 are permitted. However, the new restrictions would not apply to e-cigarettes sold exclusively in age-restricted locations (e.g., a stand-alone tobacco retailer) that either prevent minors (individuals under age 18) from entering the facility at any time, or establish a walled-off adult-only section of the facility where flavored e-cigarettes can be viewed and purchased by persons 18 and older.

Second, FDA announced that it would seek to curtail the sale of flavored e-cigarettes (other than tobacco, mint and menthol) that are sold online without "heightened age verification" processes. To advance this goal, FDA plans to identify and publish a list of best practices for online retailers [23].

Third, FDA announced that flavored cigars will no longer be subject to the extended compliance date for premarket authorization (which currently sets the premarket application deadline for cigars on the market on August 8, 2016 to be August 8, 2021). However, this policy does not apply to the entire product category, as certain flavored cigars are considered "grandfathered" and exempt from premarket review if they were on the market as of February 15, 2007, as discussed above. To address this gap in regulatory authority, FDA plans to propose a product standard that would ban all flavored cigars [23].

Fourth, FDA announced plans to publish a Proposed Rule in the Federal Register that would seek to ban menthol in combustible tobacco products, including cigarettes and cigars [23].

The Commissioner also noted that FDA plans to continue to aggressively pursue removing e-cigarettes marketed to children and/or appealing to youth from the market. These marketing practices may include "using popular children's cartoon or animated characters" or "names of products favored by kids like brands of candy or soda."

On March 13, 2019 FDA published a new draft guidance document entitled, *Modifications to Compliance Policy for Certain Deemed Tobacco Products* [24]. The draft guidance formalizes the November 2018 proposal from FDA discussed above, but makes several changes. More specifically, the draft guidance eliminates the compliance policy for flavored e-cigarettes (other than tobacco, mint, menthol and unflavored products) sold or marketed in a manner that is (a) targeted to minors or likely to promote ENDS use by minors, or (b) offered for sale in ways that pose a greater risk of minor access. Such products will be subject to immediate enforcement.

In terms of targeting minors, the guidance states that FDA is evaluating how companies may utilize social media to market to minors, as well as radio and television (which are platforms that are prohibited for cigarette advertising). FDA further implied that products with labeling and/or advertising that use "youth appealing cartoons as well as the use of minors or people who appear to be minors in multimedia advertisements" could be the subject of enforcement. The draft guidance also identifies the following circumstances which pose a "greater risks of minor access":

1. Products sold in locations that minors are able to enter at any time (e.g., the entire establishment or an area within the establishment);

2. Products sold through retail establishments and online retail locations that have sold to minors—as indicated by FDA's searchable retailer inspection database—after issuance of the final guidance document;

3. Products sold online without a limit on the quantity of product that a customer may purchase within a given period of time; or

4. Products sold online without independent, third-party age-and identity-verification services that compare customer information against third-party data sources, such as public records.

The draft guidance also shortens the compliance policy by 1 year for all flavored ENDS (other than tobacco, mint, menthol and unflavored products), even if such products are marketed responsibly to adults. If the draft guidance is finalized, such flavored products on the market on August 8, 2016 will have until August 8, 2021 to submit PMTAs (which must be accepted by FDA for substantive review).

Finally, the guidance keeps in place, for the time being, the existing compliance policy for tobacco, mint, menthol and unflavored ENDS on the market as of August 8, 2016. Accordingly, these products still have until August 8, 2022 to submit premarket applications.

FDA indicated that the reason it is modifying the compliance policy for e-cigarettes in the manner described above is (i) "to encourage more prompt filing of premarket submissions for certain ENDS products"; (ii) "to focus the Agency's enforcement resources where there is a greater threat to public health"; and (iii) "to balance that public health threat against the potential benefit to providing adult smokers noncombustible options to allow them to completely switch from the use of combustible products."

While it is unclear how FDA will enforce the new compliance policy if it becomes effective, the draft guidance expressly places the onus on manufacturers to control distribution and sale of their products to retail customers by, among other things, "requiring terms, conditions, or controls in their contracts with downstream distributors (wholesalers, distributors, importers and/or retailers) to prevent youth access."

3. Conclusion

The e-cigarette industry has grown rapidly in the United States since the products were first introduced to the market in 2007. Regulators have struggled to keep up with the evolving technology and are still grappling with the public health consequences—both pro and con. In the USA, the FDA's new authority over traditional tobacco products such as cigarettes was extended to cover e-cigarettes and other novel products. Now, newly deemed tobacco products are subject to the Tobacco Control Act requirements including, among other things, premarket authorization for new products, ingredient reporting, manufacturing establishment registration, harmful constituent testing, and sales and marketing restrictions. Regulators also continue to adopt policies and regulations to address new issues that emerge (i.e., underage use).

Manufacturers of flavored e-cigarettes should be most concerned with complying with FDA's recently revised premarket review compliance policy. In this regard, to potentially avoid being subject to immediate enforcement, and to remain eligible for the August 8, 2021 PMTA compliance date, manufacturers of flavored e-cigarettes must work with their retailers and distributors to ensure that their products are not sold in (1) all-age retailers (i.e., non-adult only facilities such as convenience stores and gas stations) that do not have separate walled-off section for flavored products, (2) online stores that do not have a limit on bulk purchases or third-party age and identity verification services, or (3) brick-and-mortar and online stores that have previously been cited for selling products to minors.

Manufacturers must further ensure that their products are not viewed as targeting or promoting use to minors. Companies should review their labeling, packaging, social media, websites, and advertising/marketing materials with the understanding that FDA could broadly argue that the use of certain flavors, descriptive flavor names, packaging and label colors, images of food, fruit, or desert, cartoon images or illustrations, playful characters, or young models, among other things, might trigger immediate enforcement under the modified compliance policy.

Finally, even if manufacturers can avoid immediate enforcement against their flavored e-cigarettes, the August 8, 2021 compliance date is fast approaching. It is critical that companies start working to prepare PMTAs sooner rather than later to have any chance of meeting that deadline.

Conflict of interest

Author Azim Chowdhury is a Partner at Keller and Heckman LLP in Washington, DC. In his law practice he represents tobacco and e-cigarettes companies in matters of regulatory compliance. He is also counsel to the Right to be Smoke-Free Coalition, a trade association of e-cigarette businesses that are challenging FDA's Deeming Rule in court.

Author details

Azim Chowdhury
Keller and Heckman LLP, Washington, DC, USA

*Address all correspondence to: chowdhury@khlaw.com

References

[1] Prior to the Tobacco Control Act, the Federal Trade Commission (FTC) had primary jurisdiction over the advertising and marketing of traditional tobacco products, such as cigarettes and smokeless tobacco

[2] Technically, the minimum purchase age, nicotine addiction warning and vending machine sale restriction only apply to deemed "covered" tobacco products, which is defined in the Deeming Rule to mean any tobacco product deemed to be subject to the Tobacco Control Act, but excludes any component or part that is not made or derived from tobacco. 21 C.F.R. § 1140.3. 2018

[3] A "finished" tobacco product is defined in the Deeming Rule as "a tobacco product, including all components and parts, sealed in final packaging intended for consumer use"

[4] FDA. Guidance for Industry: Registration and Product Listing for Owners and Operators of Domestic Tobacco Product Establishments [Internet]. 2014. Available from: http://www.fda.gov/downloads/TobaccoProducts/GuidanceComplianceRegulatoryInformation/UCM191940.pdf [Accessed: December 10, 2018]

[5] Food, Drug, and Cosmetic Act, 21 U.S.C. § 905(i)(3)

[6] Food, Drug, and Cosmetic Act, 21 U.S.C. § 905(g)

[7] Food, Drug, and Cosmetic Act, 21 U.S.C. § 704

[8] Food, Drug, and Cosmetic Act, 21 U.S.C. § 904(a)(1)-(2)

[9] For purposes of this reporting requirement, an additive means "any substance the intended use of which results or may reasonably be expected to result, directly or indirectly, in its becoming a component or otherwise affecting the characteristic of any tobacco product (including any substances intended for use as a flavoring or coloring or in producing, manufacturing, packing, processing, preparing, treating, packaging, transporting, or holding), except that such term does not include tobacco or a pesticide chemical residue in or on raw tobacco or a pesticide chemical"

[10] Food, Drug, and Cosmetic Act, 21 U.S.C. § 904(a)(3)

[11] FDA. Guidance for Industry: Listing of Ingredients in Tobacco Products (Revised)* [Internet]. 2018. Available from: https://www.fda.gov/downloads/TobaccoProducts/Labeling/RulesRegulationsGuidance/UCM527044.pdf [Accessed: December 10, 2018]

[12] FDA. Guidance for Industry: Health Document Submission Requirements for Tobacco Products (Revised)* [Internet]. 2017. Available from: https://www.fda.gov/downloads/tobaccoproducts/labeling/rulesregulationsguidance/ucm208916.pdf [Accessed: January 18, 2019]

[13] 77 Fed. Reg. 20,034 (April 3, 2012)

[14] FDA. Draft Guidance for Industry: Reporting Harmful and Potentially Harmful Constituents in Tobacco Products and Tobacco Smoke Under Section 904(a)(3) of the Federal Food, Drug, and Cosmetic Act [Internet]. 2012. Available from: http://www.fda.gov/downloads/TobaccoProducts/GuidanceComplianceRegulatoryInformation/UCM297828.pdf [Accessed: December 10, 2018]

[15] Food, Drug, and Cosmetic Act, 21 U.S.C. § 915

[16] 21 C.F.R. § 1143.3(a) (2018)

[17] 81 Fed. Reg. 28979 (May 10, 2016)

[18] Phillip Morris USA Inc., et al. v. United States Food and Drug Administration, et al., 202 F. Supp. 3d, 31 (D.D.C. 2016)

[19] 21 U.S.C. § 387j(c) (2018)

[20] On July 21, 2017, the U.S. District Court for the District of Columbia ruled in the Nicopure Labs, LLC v. Food and Drug Administration lawsuit brought by the e-cigarette industry challenging aspects of the Deeming Rule. The court ruled entirely in favor of the FDA granting the agency's motion for summary judgment and holding that: (1) FDA acted within the scope of its statutory authority; namely, that it was legally permitted to e-cigarettes as tobacco products subject to regulation; (2) it was not arbitrary and capricious for the agency to subject e-cigarettes to premarket review and labeling requirements; (3) the new rules being applied to e-cigarettes do not violate the First or the Fifth Amendments to the Constitution; and (4) the agency was not required to undertake a formal cost-benefit analysis when promulgated the Deeming Rule. That decision has been appealed to the U.S. Court of Appeals for the District of Columbia Circuit

[21] FDA. FDA Announces Comprehensive Regulatory Plan to Shift Trajectory of Tobacco-Related Disease, Death [Internet]. Available from: https://www.fda.gov/NewsEvents/Newsroom/PressAnnouncements/ucm568923.htm?utm_campaign=CTP%20News%3A%20NAS%20Report%20-%2012318&utm_medium=email&utm_source=Eloqua&elqTrackId=eee7ad075ae24d0b86dee239fd30bd01&elq=aa6a287fc5c44ef29e6f0e9b81140760&elqaid=2177&elqat=1&elqCampaignId=1520 [Accessed: December 10, 2018]

[22] FDA. FDA, Warning Letters and Civil Money Penalties Issued to Retailers for Selling JUUL and Other E-Cigarettes to Minors [Internet]. 2018. Available from: https://www.fda.gov/tobaccoproducts/newsevents/ucm605278.htm [Accessed: December 10, 2018]

[23] FDA. FDA, Statement From FDA Commissioner Scott Gottlieb, M.D., on Proposed New Steps to Protect Youth by Preventing Access to Flavored Tobacco Products and Banning Menthol in Cigarettes [Internet]. 2018. Available from: https://www.fda.gov/NewsEvents/Newsroom/PressAnnouncements/ucm625884.htm [Accessed: December 10, 2018]

[24] FDA. Draft Guidance for Industry: Modifications to Compliance Policy for Certain Deemed Tobacco Products [Internet]. 2019. Available from: https://www.fda.gov/downloads/TobaccoProducts/Labeling/RulesRegulationsGuidance/UCM633281.pdf [Accessed: April 15, 2019]

Chapter 5

Antagonism of Opioid μ Receptors for Smoking Cessation

Xiu Liu

Abstract

Opioid neurotransmission plays a role in rewarding process including the reinforcing actions of nicotine. In the past four decades, a great effort has been exercised to test the effectiveness of nonselective opioid antagonists (mainly naloxone and naltrexone) for smoking cessation. However, both clinical and animal researches have yielded equivocal results. That may be attributable to the fact that opioid receptors have three distinctive subtypes (μ, δ, and κ), functions of which are from complimentary to opposite. Our laboratory studies have used animal models of nicotine self-administration to examine involvement of individual opioid receptor subtypes in the reinforcement of nicotine. Specifically, rats were trained in daily 1-h sessions to press a lever to intravenously self-administer nicotine, and antagonists selective for the three subtypes of opioid receptors were administered prior to the test sessions. Results showed that selective blockade of the μ, but not δ or κ, opioid receptors effectively reduced nicotine self-administration, whereas it produced no effect on food self-administration. These results indicate that activation of the opioid μ, but not δ or κ, receptors is specifically involved in nicotine reinforcement. It is suggested that opioid μ receptor-mediated neurotransmission would be a promising target for developing smoking cessation medication.

Keywords: nicotine self-administration, opioid receptors, smoking cessation

1. Introduction

Tobacco-related diseases are a major problem in many perspectives from human health to social economics [1]. For example, in the United States, tobacco smoking becomes a leading cause of death, accounting for the loss of 480,000 lives each year. Alarmingly, every day more than 3200 youth aged 18 years or younger smoke their first cigarette, and 2100 young people become daily cigarette smokers. The prevalence rates of smoking are 7.2% in middle and 20.2% in high school, accounting for a total young smokers being about 4 million [2]. Although almost all smokers want to quit smoking and make attempts, up to 97% of them relapse to tobacco smoking [3–6]. Unfortunately, the currently available medications, i.e., nicotine replacement, bupropion, and varenicline, show low clinical effectiveness [7–11].

Opioid neurotransmission has been implicated in mediating rewarding actions and dependence of drugs of abuse including nicotine [12–16]. For instance, nicotine administration has been found to increase expression and release of opioid peptides in mesolimbic regions [17–22]. Opioid receptor antagonists have been reported to decrease nicotine-induced dopamine release in the nucleus accumbens, an important terminal region of the mesolimbic dopamine circuitry [23], reduce nicotine reward [24, 25], and precipitate withdrawal symptoms in rats treated chronically with nicotine [26].

Over the past four decades or so, however, clinical effort to test the potential of opioid antagonists (mainly naloxone and naltrexone) for smoking cessation has yielded equivocal results: some trials reported that these antagonists reduced consumption of cigarettes, while others failed to find any benefit [27–37]. Similarly, laboratory animal research has also produced mixed findings. In our own studies, neither acute nor chronic pretreatment with naltrexone across seven daily nicotine self-administration test sessions altered nicotine intake in the rats trained to steadily self-administer nicotine [38]. That is consistent with previous reports showing that naloxone and naltrexone did not produce an effect on nicotine self-administration [39, 40]. However, intracranial manipulation studies have found that a μ-opioid agonist, DAMGO, microinjected into the ventral tegmental area [41] or the pedunculopontine tegmental nucleus [42] effectively reduced nicotine self-administration in rats. Studies using knockout mice showed that deletion of the μ-opioid receptors or their endogenous ligand β-endorphin resulted in decreased rewarding properties of nicotine as measured by the conditioned place preference paradigm [43, 44]. Moreover, a recent rat study reported that naloxone reduced nicotine self-administration [45].

These inconsistent results in both clinical and animal research may be attributable to the existence of different subtypes of the opioid receptors. There are three main subtypes of the opioid receptors: μ, δ, and κ [46–48]. These receptors have quite divergent and in some cases even opposite actions. In the drug rewarding processes, for instance, activation of the μ and κ receptors may have opposite actions with the κ receptors opposing rewarding actions and/or enhancing aversive effects of drugs [49–52]. In knockout mice, animals deficient in μ receptors showed decreased level of anxiety, whereas the δ receptor knockout mice had higher anxiety [53], suggesting these two subtypes have an opposite role in regulating anxiety states. In the tests measuring the anxiety states induced by nicotine, the μ and δ receptor antagonism produced opposite effects, whereas the κ receptor antagonist showed no effect [54]. Therefore, due to their broad spectrum of actions, the nonselective receptor antagonists such as naloxone and naltrexone can block different opioid receptors, and unfortunately the effects of blocking individual types of receptors might have offset one another.

2. Research purposes

In light of the facts that nonselective antagonism of opioid receptors produced inconclusive results for smoking cessation, that three subtypes of opioid receptors exist with distinct and even opposing functions, and that effects of antagonizing these individual receptor subtypes have received little experimental attention, it is imperative to elucidate the involvement of the opioid receptor subtypes in mediating nicotine reinforcement. Thus, our laboratory used animal models of tobacco smoking and the currently available antagonists that are highly selective for the different subtypes of the opioid receptors to examine the roles of the μ, δ, and κ receptors in nicotine consumption behavior [55].

3. Experimental procedures

Male Sprague-Dawley rats (n = 26) were trained in daily 1-h sessions to intravenously self-administer nicotine (0.03 mg/kg/infusion, free base) after implantation of an indwelling intravenous catheter under isoflurane anesthesia. In each session, animals were placed in the standard operant conditioning chambers and connected to the drug delivery system. The sessions were initiated by introduction of two levers. Once responses on the active lever met a fixed-ratio 5 requirement, an infusion of nicotine was dispensed with a presentation of an auditory/visual stimulus consisting of a 5 s tone and 20 s turn-on of the lever light. All rats received 25 daily self-administration training sessions before any pharmacological tests because our work showed that rats readily developed stable nicotine self-administration behavior within 25 sessions [56].

4. Main research findings

Blockade of the μ opioid receptors by a selective antagonist naloxonazine dose-dependently reduced lever-press responses and correspondingly the number of nicotine infusions rats willingly self-administered. However, naloxonazine did not alter food self-administering responses, which was tested in the same set of rats that were retrained for food self-administration after completion of nicotine test. In contrast, neither did blockade of the δ receptors via administration of the selective antagonist naltrindole nor the κ-selective antagonist 5′-guanidinonaltrindole (GNTI) change nicotine self-administration behavior (**Figure 1**).

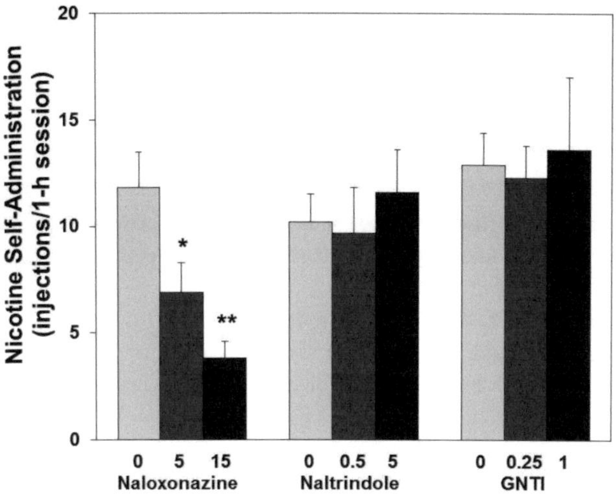

Figure 1.
*Effects of antagonists selective for μ (naloxonazine), δ (naltrindole), and κ (GNTI) receptors on nicotine self-administration in rats. The doses of these antagonists are in mg/kg. Nicotine self-administration data are expressed as mean (±SEM). *$p < 0.05$, **$P < 0.01$ significant difference from respective 0 (vehicle) condition.*

5. Discussion

The significant finding is that naloxonazine produced a specific suppressant effect on the lever-press responses maintained by nicotine self-administration, i.e., the primary reinforcement of nicotine. Given that naloxonazine did not change food self-administering responses, indicating no nonspecific interference with operant behavior directed to get natural reward, the results indicate the critical involvement of opioid neurotransmission via the μ receptors in the nicotine rewarding process. The underlying mechanism may involve the μ modulation of dopamine neurons in the mesolimbic circuitry, which mediates the rewarding properties of drug of abuse including nicotine. For example, in the ventral tegmental area, opioid peptides modulate dopamine neurotransmission predominantly via activation of the μ receptors [23], and in the nucleus accumbens, μ agonist inhibited dopamine overflow, and this effect was reversed by naloxonazine [57]. The suppressant effect of naloxonazine on nicotine intake is in line with previous research suggesting a role of the μ receptors in mediating the reinforcement of nicotine and tobacco smoking [27, 31, 35, 43–45]. Of significance is that our results further pinpoint the μ subtype of the opioid receptors in mediating reinforcement of nicotine. Therefore, these findings lend support for the continued clinical effort to test the effectiveness of opioid antagonists for smoking cessation and further instructively suggest that the effort focus should be shifted to targeting at the μ receptors.

The finding that naltrindole produced no effect on nicotine intake indicates that opioid neurotransmission via the δ receptors may not mediate the reinforcing actions of nicotine as measured by the operant nicotine self-administration paradigm. It is in line with evidence showing that this agent produced no change in nicotine-induced sensitization [58] and consistent with another report showing unaltered nicotine intake after naltrindole pretreatment using similar nicotine self-administration procedures [45]. However, these negative results seem to be at odds with a previous study using knockout mice that were deficient of preproenkephalin gene (producing enkephalin, the endogenous agonist for the δ receptors). These knockout mice showed a significant decrease in nicotine-induced conditioned place preference, indicating a reduction of the rewarding effects of nicotine [59]. This discrepancy regarding involvement of the δ receptors in nicotine reward may be attributable to the significant differences in subjects (rats versus gene knockout mice) and the methods of measuring nicotine reward (self-administration versus conditioned place preference). Besides, it is interesting to note the evidence showing that the δ receptors have been implicated in other actions of nicotine. For instance, the δ receptor antagonists were reported to change nicotine-induced antinociception [60] and anxiogenic response [54]. Nevertheless, an alternative explanation of the knockout mouse data exists. Due to the fact that in addition to preferentially activating the δ receptors enkephalin also acts at the μ receptors [61], it is argued that the reduced rewarding actions of nicotine in these knockout mice may result at least to some extent from the diminished μ receptor activities. Thus, the results obtained from these knockout mice in fact reconcile with the suppression of nicotine self-administration by naloxonazine observed in our study.

There was no effect of κ-selective antagonist 5′-guanidinonaltrindole (GNTI) on nicotine self-administration. This finding is consistent with results obtained from gene knockout mice. In the mice deficient of prodynorphin genes, which produce dynorphin, the endogenous agonist for k receptors, the conditioned place preference induced by nicotine (and ethanol and cocaine as well) was comparable to that observed in their wild-type counterparts [51, 62, 63]. In another report [45], however, the elevated activation of the κ receptors by experimenter administered agonist seemed to interfere with operant behavior for nicotine intake. In that study [45], the selective κ receptor agonist U50,488 changed nicotine self-administering behavior in opposing directions depending on the doses administered. An increase of nicotine self-administration was observed after pretreatment with a low dose of 0.3 mg/kg, whereas rats decreased their nicotine self-administration after administration of higher doses (1 and 3 mg/kg). It should be noted that U50,488 was found to produce "abnormal" behaviors (such as biting the edge of behavioral testing arena) at doses above 0.9 mg/kg [64] and that the κ agonists may bind to other opioid receptors and thereby to produce opposing actions [65]. Furthermore, it is interesting to note that activation of the κ receptors may play a role in the increased drug self-administration in drug-dependent but not non-dependent subjects [66, 67]. For instance, nor-BNI (a κ receptor antagonist) has been found to effectively reduce the escalated cocaine self-administration in rats with a prolonged access to cocaine and the increased ethanol intake in rats that became ethanol dependent by an ethanol vapor inhalation procedure [67, 68].

6. Conclusions

These research results demonstrate that nicotine self-administration behavior is sensitive to pharmacological antagonism of the μ, but not the δ or the κ, opioid receptors. Together with the evidence showing that nicotine administration enhances release of the endogenous μ receptor ligand endorphin [19, 69–71], these data indicate a critical role of opioid neurotransmission via the μ receptors in the rewarding properties of nicotine. On one hand, these results help understand the inconsistent outcomes obtained from bot clinical trials and animal tests using the nonselective antagonists naloxone and naltrexone. On the other hand, the findings suggest that focusing on manipulation of the μ receptor-mediated pathways within the opioid system might prove to be a fruitful strategy for the development of medication for nicotine addiction and smoking cessation.

Acknowledgements

The research work reviewed in this chapter was supported by NIH grants R01 DA017288 and R01 DA037277 from the National Institute on Drug Abuse as well as the State of California Tobacco-Related Disease Research Program grant #12KT-0188. The authors would like to thank Courtney Jernigan, Lisa Biswas, Erin Harrison, Ramachandram Avusula, Thomas Rousselle, and Thuy Tran for their excellent technical assistance.

Author details

Xiu Liu
Department of Pathology, University of Mississippi Medical Center, Jackson, MS, USA

*Address all correspondence to: xliu@umc.edu

References

[1] WHO. 2015. Available from: https://www.who.int/news-room/fact-sheets/detail/tobacco

[2] CDC. Tobacco use among middle and high school students—United States, 2011-2016. Morbidity and Mortality Weekly Report. 2017;**66**(23): 597-603

[3] Benowitz NL. Nicotine addiction. *The New England Journal of Medicine*. 2010;**362**(24):2295-2303

[4] Shiffman S, Mason KM, Henningfield JE. Tobacco dependence treatments: Review and prospectus. Annual Review of Public Health. 1998;**19**:335-358

[5] Hughes JR, Keely J, Naud S. Shape of the relapse curve and long-term abstinence among untreated smokers. Addiction. 2004;**99**(1):29-38

[6] CDC. Current cigarette smoking among adults—United States. Morbidity and Mortality Weekly Report. 2014;**63**:29-34

[7] Jorenby DE, Hays JT, Rigotti NA, Azoulay S, Watsky EJ, Williams KE, et al. Efficacy of varenicline, an alpha4beta2 nicotinic acetylcholine receptor partial agonist, vs placebo or sustained-release bupropion for smoking cessation: A randomized controlled trial. JAMA. 2006;**296**(1):56-63

[8] Gonzales D, Rennard SI, Nides M, Oncken C, Azoulay S, Billing CB, et al. Varenicline, an alpha4beta2 nicotinic acetylcholine receptor partial agonist, vs sustained-release bupropion and placebo for smoking cessation: A randomized controlled trial. JAMA. 2006;**296**(1):47-55

[9] Aubin HJ, Bobak A, Britton JR, Oncken C, Billing CB Jr, Gong J, et al. Varenicline versus transdermal nicotine patch for smoking cessation: Results from a randomised, open-label trial. Thorax. 2008;**63**(8):717-724

[10] Vogeler T, McClain C, Evoy KE. Combination bupropion sr and varenicline for smoking cessation: A systematic review. The American Journal of Drug and Alcohol Abuse. 2016;**42**(2):129-139

[11] Rose JE, Behm FM. Combination treatment with varenicline and bupropion in an adaptive smoking cessation paradigm. The American Journal of Psychiatry. 2014;**171**(11):1199-1205

[12] Gianoulakis C. Endogenous opioids and addiction to alcohol and other drugs of abuse. Current Topics in Medicinal Chemistry. 2004;**4**(1):39-50

[13] Pomerleau OF. Endogenous opioids and smoking: A review of progress and problems. Psychoneuroendocrinology. 1998;**23**(2):115-130

[14] Xue Y, Domino EF. Tobacco/nicotine and endogenous brain opioids. Progress in Neuro-Psychopharmacology and Biological Psychiatry. 2008;**32**(5): 1131-1138

[15] Le Merrer J, Becker JA, Befort K, Kieffer BL. Reward processing by the opioid system in the brain. Physiological Reviews. 2009;**89**(4):1379-1412

[16] Berrendero F, Robledo P, Trigo JM, Martin-Garcia E, Maldonado R. Neurobiological mechanisms involved in nicotine dependence and reward: Participation of the endogenous opioid system. Neuroscience and Biobehavioral Reviews. 2010;**35**(2):220-231

[17] Houdi AA, Dasgupta R, Kindy MS. Effect of nicotine use and

withdrawal on brain preproenkephalin a mRNA. Brain Research. 1998;**799**(2): 257-263

[18] Houdi AA, Pierzchala K, Marson L, Palkovits M, Van Loon GR. Nicotine-induced alteration in Tyr-Gly-Gly and Met-enkephalin in discrete brain nuclei reflects altered enkephalin neuron activity. Peptides. 1991;**12**(1):161-166

[19] Boyadjieva NI, Sarkar DK. The secretory response of hypothalamic beta-endorphin neurons to acute and chronic nicotine treatments and following nicotine withdrawal. Life Sciences. 1997;**61**(6):PL59-PL66

[20] Davenport KE, Houdi AA, Van Loon GR. Nicotine protects against mu-opioid receptor antagonism by beta-funaltrexamine: Evidence for nicotine-induced release of endogenous opioids in brain. Neuroscience Letters. 1990;**113**(1):40-46

[21] Dhatt RK, Gudehithlu KP, Wemlinger TA, Tejwani GA, Neff NH, Hadjiconstantinou M. Preproenkephalin mRNA and methionine-enkephalin content are increased in mouse striatum after treatment with nicotine. Journal of Neurochemistry. 1995;**64**(4):1878-1883

[22] Pierzchala K, Houdi AA, Van Loon GR. Nicotine-induced alterations in brain regional concentrations of native and cryptic Met- and Leu-enkephalin. Peptides. 1987;**8**(6):1035-1043

[23] Tanda G, Di Chiara G. A dopamine-mu1 opioid link in the rat ventral tegmentum shared by palatable food (Fonzies) and non-psychostimulant drugs of abuse. The European Journal of Neuroscience. 1998;**10**(3):1179-1187

[24] Walters CL, Cleck JN, Kuo YC, Blendy JA. Mu-opioid receptor and creb activation are required for nicotine reward. Neuron. 2005;**46**(6):933-943

[25] Zarrindast MR, Faraji N, Rostami P, Sahraei H, Ghoshouni H. Cross-tolerance between morphine- and nicotine-induced conditioned place preference in mice. Pharmacology, Biochemistry, and Behavior. 2003;**74**(2):363-369

[26] Malin DH, Lake JR, Carter VA, Cunningham JS, Wilson OB. Naloxone precipitates nicotine abstinence syndrome in the rat. Psychopharmacology. 1993;**112**(2-3):339-342

[27] Karras A, Kane JM. Naloxone reduces cigarette smoking. Life Sciences. 1980;**27**(17):1541-1545

[28] Nemeth-Coslett R, Griffiths RR. Naloxone does not affect cigarette smoking. Psychopharmacology. 1986;**89**(3):261-264

[29] Gorelick DA, Rose J, Jarvik ME. Effect of naloxone on cigarette smoking. Journal of Substance Abuse. 1988;**1**(2):153-159

[30] Krishnan-Sarin S, Rosen MI, O'Malley SS. Naloxone challenge in smokers. Preliminary evidence of an opioid component in nicotine dependence. Archives of General Psychiatry. 1999;**56**(7):663-668

[31] King AC, Meyer PJ. Naltrexone alteration of acute smoking response in nicotine-dependent subjects. Pharmacology, Biochemistry, and Behavior. 2000;**66**(3):563-572

[32] Sutherland G, Stapleton JA, Russell MA, Feyerabend C. Naltrexone, smoking behaviour and cigarette withdrawal. Psychopharmacology. 1995;**120**(4):418-425

[33] Wong GY, Wolter TD, Croghan GA, Croghan IT, Offord KP, Hurt RD. A randomized trial of naltrexone for smoking cessation. Addiction. 1999;**94**(8):1227-1237

[34] King A, de Wit H, Riley RC, Cao D, Niaura R, Hatsukami D. Efficacy of naltrexone in smoking cessation: A preliminary study and an examination of sex differences. Nicotine & Tobacco Research. 2006;**8**(5):671-682

[35] Rukstalis M, Jepson C, Strasser A, Lynch KG, Perkins K, Patterson F, et al. Naltrexone reduces the relative reinforcing value of nicotine in a cigarette smoking choice paradigm. Psychopharmacology. 2005;**180**(1):41-48

[36] Ray R, Jepson C, Patterson F, Strasser A, Rukstalis M, Perkins K, et al. Association of OPRM1 A118G variant with the relative reinforcing value of nicotine. Psychopharmacology. 2006;**188**(3):355-363

[37] Wewers ME, Dhatt R, Tejwani GA. Naltrexone administration affects ad libitum smoking behavior. Psychopharmacology. 1998;**140**(2):185-190

[38] Liu X, Palmatier MI, Caggiula AR, Sved AF, Donny EC, Gharib M, et al. Naltrexone attenuation of conditioned but not primary reinforcement of nicotine in rats. Psychopharmacology. 2009;**202**(4):589-598

[39] Corrigall WA, Coen KM. Opiate antagonists reduce cocaine but not nicotine self-administration. Psychopharmacology. 1991;**104**(2):167-170

[40] DeNoble VJ, Mele PC. Intravenous nicotine self-administration in rats: Effects of mecamylamine, hexamethonium and naloxone. Psychopharmacology. 2006;**184**(3-4):266-272

[41] Corrigall WA, Coen KM, Adamson KL, Chow BL, Zhang J. Response of nicotine self-administration in the rat to manipulations of mu-opioid and gamma-aminobutyric acid receptors in the ventral tegmental area. Psychopharmacology. 2000;**149**(2):107-114

[42] Corrigall WA, Coen KM, Zhang J, Adamson L. Pharmacological manipulations of the pedunculopontine tegmental nucleus in the rat reduce self-administration of both nicotine and cocaine. Psychopharmacology. 2002;**160**(2):198-205

[43] Berrendero F, Kieffer BL, Maldonado R. Attenuation of nicotine-induced antinociception, rewarding effects, and dependence in mu-opioid receptor knock-out mice. The Journal of Neuroscience. 2002;**22**(24):10935-10940

[44] Trigo JM, Zimmer A, Maldonado R. Nicotine anxiogenic and rewarding effects are decreased in mice lacking beta-endorphin. Neuropharmacology. 2009;**56**(8):1147-1153

[45] Ismayilova N, Shoaib M. Alteration of intravenous nicotine self-administration by opioid receptor agonist and antagonists in rats. Psychopharmacology. 2010;**210**(2):211-220

[46] Snyder SH, Pasternak GW. Historical review: Opioid receptors. Trends in Pharmacological Sciences. 2003;**24**(4):198-205

[47] Dhawan BN, Cesselin F, Raghubir R, Reisine T, Bradley PB, Portoghese PS, et al. International Union of Pharmacology. XII. Classification of opioid receptors. Pharmacological Reviews. 1996;**48**(4):567-592

[48] Mansour A, Fox CA, Akil H, Watson SJ. Opioid-receptor mRNA expression in the rat cns: Anatomical and functional implications. Trends in Neurosciences. 1995;**18**(1):22-29

[49] Shippenberg TS, Zapata A, Chefer VI. Dynorphin and the pathophysiology of drug addiction. Pharmacology & Therapeutics. 2007;**116**(2):306-321

[50] Hasebe K, Kawai K, Suzuki T, Kawamura K, Tanaka T, Narita M, et al. Possible pharmacotherapy of the opioid kappa receptor agonist for drug dependence. Annals of the New York Academy of Sciences. 2004;**1025**:404-413

[51] Galeote L, Berrendero F, Bura SA, Zimmer A, Maldonado R. Prodynorphin gene disruption increases the sensitivity to nicotine self-administration in mice. International Journal of Neuropsychopharmacology. 2009;**12**(5):615-625

[52] Matsuzawa S, Suzuki T, Misawa M, Nagase H. Different roles of mu-, delta- and kappa-opioid receptors in ethanol-associated place preference in rats exposed to conditioned fear stress. European Journal of Pharmacology. 1999;**368**(1):9-16

[53] Filliol D, Ghozland S, Chluba J, Martin M, Matthes HW, Simonin F, et al. Mice deficient for delta- and mu-opioid receptors exhibit opposing alterations of emotional responses. Nature Genetics. 2000;**25**(2):195-200

[54] Balerio GN, Aso E, Maldonado R. Involvement of the opioid system in the effects induced by nicotine on anxiety-like behaviour in mice. Psychopharmacology. 2005;**181**(2):260-269

[55] Liu X, Jernigan C. Activation of the opioid mu1, but not delta or kappa, receptors is required for nicotine reinforcement in a rat model of drug self-administration. Progress in Neuro-Psychopharmacology and Biological Psychiatry. 2011;**35**(1):146-153

[56] Liu X, Caggiula AR, Yee SK, Nobuta H, Poland RE, Pechnick RN. Reinstatement of nicotine-seeking behavior by drug-associated stimuli after extinction in rats. Psychopharmacology. 2006;**184**(3-4):417-425

[57] Britt JP, McGehee DS. Presynaptic opioid and nicotinic receptor modulation of dopamine overflow in the nucleus accumbens. The Journal of Neuroscience. 2008;**28**(7):1672-1681

[58] Heidbreder C, Shoaib M, Shippenberg TS. Differential role of delta-opioid receptors in the development and expression of behavioral sensitization to cocaine. European Journal of Pharmacology. 1996;**298**(3):207-216

[59] Berrendero F, Mendizabal V, Robledo P, Galeote L, Bilkei-Gorzo A, Zimmer A, et al. Nicotine-induced antinociception, rewarding effects, and physical dependence are decreased in mice lacking the preproenkephalin gene. The Journal of Neuroscience. 2005;**25**(5):1103-1112

[60] Campbell VC, Taylor RE, Tizabi Y. Effects of selective opioid receptor antagonists on alcohol-induced and nicotine-induced antinociception. Alcoholism, Clinical and Experimental Research. 2007;**31**(8):1435-1440

[61] Drake CT, Chavkin C, Milner TA. Opioid systems in the dentate gyrus. Progress in Brain Research. 2007;**163**:245-263

[62] Blednov YA, Walker D, Martinez M, Harris RA. Reduced alcohol consumption in mice lacking preprodynorphin. Alcohol. 2006;**40**(2):73-86

[63] McLaughlin JP, Marton-Popovici M, Chavkin C. Kappa opioid receptor antagonism and prodynorphin gene disruption block stress-induced behavioral responses. The Journal of Neuroscience. 2003;**23**(13):5674-5683

[64] Kitamura T, Ogawa M, Yamada Y. The individual and combined effects of U50,488, and flurbiprofen axetil on visceral pain in conscious rats. Anesthesia and Analgesia. 2009;**108**(6):1964-1966

[65] Heidbreder CA, Babovic-Vuksanovic D, Shoaib M, Shippenberg TS. Development of behavioral sensitization to cocaine: Influence of kappa opioid receptor agonists. The Journal of Pharmacology and Experimental Therapeutics. 1995;**275**(1):150-163

[66] Glick S, Maisonneuve I, Raucci J, Archer S. Kappa opioid inhibition on morphine and cocaine self-administration on rats. Brain Research. 1995;**681**(1-2):147-152

[67] Wee S, Orio L, Ghirmai S, Cashman JR, Koob GF. Inhibition of kappa opioid receptors attenuated increased cocaine intake in rats with extended access to cocaine. Psychopharmacology. 2009;**205**(4):565-575

[68] Walker BM, Zorrilla EP, Koob GF. Systemic kappa-opioid receptor antagonism by nor-binaltorphimine reduces dependence-induced excessive alcohol self-administration in rats. Addiction Biology. 2010;**16**(1):116-119

[69] Conte-Devolx B, Oliver C, Giraud P, Gillioz P, Castanas E, Lissitzky JC, et al. Effect of nicotine on in vivo secretion of melanocorticotropic hormones in the rat. Life Sciences. 1981;**28**(9):1067-1073

[70] Rosecrans JA, Hendry JS, Hong JS. Biphasic effects of chronic nicotine treatment on hypothalamic immunoreactive beta-endorphin in the mouse. Pharmacology, Biochemistry, and Behavior. 1985;**23**(1):141-143

[71] Marty MA, Erwin VG, Cornell K, Zgombick JM. Effects of nicotine on beta-endorphin, alpha MSH, and ACTH secretion by isolated perfused mouse brains and pituitary glands, in vitro. Pharmacology, Biochemistry, and Behavior. 1985;**22**(2):317-325